HEALTHY
EYES
BETTER
VISION

HEALTHY EYES BETTER VISION

EVERYDAY EYE CARE FOR THE WHOLE FAMILY

by Dr. Jeffrey Anshel

❧ **THE BODY PRESS**
a division of
PRICE STERN SLOAN
Los Angeles

© 1990 by Jeffrey Anshel
Published by The Body Press, a division of Price Stern Sloan, Inc.
360 North La Cienega Boulevard, Los Angeles, California 90048
Printed in U.S.A.
987654321

Book produced by
Summerlin Publishing Group,
P.O. Box 32012, Tucson Arizona, 85751-2012

Library of Congress Cataloging-in-Publication Data

Anshel, Jeffrey.
    Healthy eyes, better vision / by Jeffrey Anshel.
        p. cm.
    Includes bibliographical references.
    1. Eye—Care and hygiene.   2. Eye—Diseases and defects—
Popular works.   I. Title.
RE51.A63   1990   90-531
617.7—dc20   CIP

All information in this book is given without guarantees on the part of the author, contributors, consultants, producer or publisher. This book is intended only as a general guide for eye care and is not a substitute for sound diagnosis, advice or treatment from an optometrist or medical doctor. Only an optometrist or medical doctor can properly diagnose eye prob-lems and prescribe eyeglasses or other treatments. Final deci-sions about eye care must be made by each individual in con-sultation with his or her doctor. The author, contributors, consultants, producer and publisher disclaim all liability in connection with the implementation of this information.

Recognizing the importance of preserving that which has been written, Price Stern Sloan, Inc. has decided to print this book on acid-free paper.

This book is dedicated to the memory of my mother, Rochelle, whose support guided me through the most difficult of times, and to my father, Bernard, whose encouragement and faith inspires me to succeed.

Acknowledgments

I would like to acknowledge the late Dr. E.R. "Ernie" Tennant, O.D., and Dr. Hyman Wodis, O.D., whose fascination with the art and science of optometry and the world of vision opened my eyes and those of so many of my colleagues.

Thank you to Liz Burke, a great receptionist and a committed typist, who devoted so much extra time to keeping the manuscript alive.

My sincere thanks and acknowledgment to Selina, whose love and friendship through the years has always inspired me. And, of course, to my son Casey, who teaches me the real meaning of love.

I would also like to acknowledge my agent and friend, Julie Castiglia, for her commitment to this project and for sharing her ideas and friendship.

Thank you, Maggie Wahl, for magically transforming my thoughts and ideas into reality, and for being on my team.

And most of all to my lovely Elaine, whose commitment to me and our life together makes it all worthwhile.

Contents

Introduction

You may never have thought about how easy it is for you to read the words on this page. That's because your eyes are probably handling the job pretty well. Consider the fact that over 80 percent of what you learn comes in through your eyes. That says a lot about the importance of vision in learning. You may be one of the 42 percent of Americans who doesn't wear corrective lenses—if so, congratulations. That doesn't mean, though, that you don't have a vision-related problem. More than likely, you're one of the ninety million Americans who is overdue for an eye examination.

The act of seeing may seem automatic for you, so taking your eyes for granted is an easy thing to do. We're born with two eyes that, for the most part, are fully functional at birth. However, the complex function of vision, which involves the processing and understanding of visual input, requires learning. This learning happens over the first decade of life, and if it doesn't happen, a child's development will be impaired. We are mostly visually directed creatures, and our eyes are our most important connection with our world.

Vision problems are often not painful and are usually slow to develop. Many of the problems that occur are preventable—not just by reading letters on a chart once every four years or eating a lot of carrots, but by taking a little extra time to learn about your eyes and how they work for you. Signs of a vision problem may start as an occasional blur or a dull headache after reading for a short period of time. Or, you may have trouble seeing distant objects like road signs. You may feel a bit of burning or dryness in your eyes at various times. Or, you may notice that your eyes look different from their usual appearance in the bathroom mirror. Fortunately, even if something does go wrong, you can usually correct the problem if you get help soon. There is such a thing as preventive eye care, and it's easier than you may think.

This book isn't going to prevent all your vision problems. And you *won't* learn that by doing some simple exercises you'll be able to throw away your glasses, although advertising for that concept is popular these days. But by being aware of your eyes and the messages they send, you may be able to keep yourself from becoming stuck behind glasses for the rest of your life—or at least from needing a stronger prescription every year. And, you may be able to prevent serious eye damage or loss of vision.

It's a lot easier to prevent eye problems than it is to try to reverse changes that have already taken place.

If you wear glasses, there's a lot you should know about them. And, you might as well get glasses that will enhance, rather than detract from, your appearance. Contact lenses are especially complicated and should be treated more like the medical devices that they are rather than as cosmetics.

Whether you wear corrective lenses or not, you should have enough knowledge about your vision to know when to see your eye doctor—and what kind of eye doctor to see. Studies continue to show that many people don't know whether their eye-care professional is an optometrist, an optician or an ophthalmologist. And exactly what is the difference between them anyway?

The information in this book should answer most of the questions you've had about your eyes and the way you see things. I've tried to put it all in terms that are simple to understand yet still complete enough to let you know how your vision works. My hope is that this book will open your eyes to the world of vision and enable you to learn enough about your eyes so you can talk intelligently to your doctor about your vision problems. I also hope to dispel some myths about what's good for your eyes and what isn't. Here's looking at you!

CHAPTER 1

A Do-It-Yourself Basic Eye Check

I'd like to introduce you to a part of your body that you don't see very much—your eyes. Since you're always seeing *with* them, you don't often get a chance to look *at* them. You've got two fascinating organs in your body that are available for you to observe, and I hope you'll get to know them well. So get ready—you're about to start a fascinating trip into the world of vision.

LOOK AT YOUR EYES

The first thing you'll need is a mirror. Make sure you're able to get close because you'll want to be able to see some small details. A small magnifying glass will come in handy. Another good thing to have is a flashlight. A tiny one (sometimes called a "penlight") can easily fit between you and the mirror. Any good bright light will do.

Now, stand in front of the mirror and look at your eyes. They should be symmetrical. Look at how far your upper eyelids come down over your eyes. They should both come down to about the same point on each eye. Check to see if one eye is actually higher than the other. Having droopy eyelids or one eye higher than the other can be perfectly normal, but can also indicate a nerve or muscle problem or a thyroid disorder. If you've noticed a recent change in how your eyes look, I'd check with your doctor.

Notice the bone formation around your eyes. The *orbit*, the bony ridge surrounding the eye, is specifically designed to

protect the eyes, especially from foreign objects that may accidentally fly your way. Eyes that are deeply recessed into their
orbits are called "deep-set." Notice your eyelashes. The upper lid
has longer lashes and more of them. These are also designed to
protect your eye from foreign matter.

Move a little closer to the mirror and take a look at your
eyeball. The most obvious thing you'll notice is the color. This
part is called the *iris* (EYE-ris), which means rainbow, and it is
protected by a clear dome called the *cornea* (KOR-nee-ah). Shining the light directly at your eye will give you the best view of
the actual color of your eye. Colors vary from chocolate brown
to sky blue. Eyes that seem to change color from one day to the
next usually appear different due to the change in surrounding
illumination.

If you look closely at your iris you'll see that it isn't a solid col-
or but almost weblike in nature with various colors scattered
throughout. Use your magnifying glass to see this detail. Hold
the magnifying lens up near the mirror and move your head
back and forth until you get a clear image. Shine the light from
your other hand and you should see more detail. I'll talk more
about the iris later.

You may have also noticed something interesting when you
shined the light into your eye: The iris moved! This movement
caused the black spot in the middle of your eye to get smaller.
This black spot is actually a hole called the *pupil*. It is through
the pupil that light enters the eye. Check and see if both pupils
are about the same size and that they both get smaller when you
shine the light into either eye. A difference in pupil reaction is
common following head or eye injuries. It occasionally occurs as
a normal phenomenon.

ARE YOUR EYES RED?

While you're still at the mirror, pull down a lower eyelid and
take a close look at the inner side of it along with the white part
of your eye. What you are looking at is called the *conjunctiva*
(kahn-junk-TYE-vah). The conjunctiva is a *mucous membrane*,
a thin layer of tissue that secretes mucus. It lines the eyelids and
the part of the eyeball not covered by the cornea. It has an important role in keeping your eyes moist, which in turn keeps
them clear, allowing normal eyesight. The conjunctiva needs a
good blood and tear supply to do its job, so notice the tiny blood

vessels. They are very normal. Now take a look at your other inner eyelid. Also take a close look at some friends' inner eyelids. You may notice that some eyes have more blood vessels than others. This variation is normal.

The white part of your eye, the *sclera* (SKLER-ah), is the protective covering of the eye and doesn't require much of a blood supply. It's the membrane covering the sclera, the conjunctiva, that has most of the blood vessels in it. To tell if the blood vessels you see are in the conjunctiva or the sclera, simply pull the corner of your eyelid off to one side while watching closely in the mirror. The conjunctiva, which is attached to the eyelids, will move and so will its blood vessels. This movement will be slight, so look closely. If the vessels *don't* move, they are in the sclera. (A few small vessels in the sclera can also be very normal.)

If you find your eyelids and conjunctiva are very red and maybe itchy at times, you may have *conjunctivitis*, an inflammation of the conjunctiva caused by infection, allergy or irritation (see *Conjunctivitis*, page 219). People commonly use the word *pinkeye* to describe the kind of conjunctivitis caused by infection. Any irritation of your eyes should be checked professionally because there are some very serious problems that may appear mild at first. *Don't* try over-the-counter eye drops or eye "whiteners" (eye drops that promise to remove redness from the eyes); they'll only cover up your symptoms and not solve any problems.

WHAT DOES '20/20' REALLY MEAN?

Recall the last time you visited your eye doctor's office. You probably got a full examination, had what seemed like a hundred different tests, and you asked: "How are my eyes?" The answer could have been: "You have 20/20 vision!" You then walked out of the office satisfied that your eyes were in good shape. But are they? What is 20/20, and what does it mean? What is so magical about those numbers that relieves the most worried minds? Well, here's the straight scoop on the magic numbers.

First, what do the numbers mean? They are a notation that relates to the *resolving power* of the eye. *Resolving power* means how sharp your sight is, which we can define as your ability to distinguish two points from each other and not see them as just one point.

If your vision is 20/20, it means that you're seeing at twenty feet what the "optically normal" eye can see at twenty feet — that is, that your eyes can distinguish one point from another on a specific line from a standard eye chart placed twenty feet away. The chart is called a *Snellen chart,* and you'll find one on pages 5 through 8. If your vision is, let's say, 20/40, it means that you can see at twenty feet what the normal eye can see at forty feet (you have to be closer). And, if your vision is 20/100, you must be at twenty feet while the normal eye can be a hundred feet away and see the same thing as clearly. In short, the larger the bottom number is, the poorer your resolving power, which is also known as your *visual acuity.* Visual acuity is measured for distance and near vision. So now you know that 20/20 is something like a grading of eyesight.

Test Your Distance-Vision Acuity

OK, time to test how well you see. The first thing you'll need is twenty feet of space and the eye chart on pages 5 through 8. You'll need a friend to hold the book open for you and check your answers.

Start reading the chart with one eye covered, but not closed, and start with the bigger letters. Squinting is not allowed here! Continue reading line by line and have your friend keep score. The smallest line that you can comfortably read is your visual acuity. Now test the other eye.

The Snellen chart is only one test for visual acuity, and in any case, no real significance should be placed on visual acuity alone. As a matter of fact, even if you read the 20/20 line perfectly, you still may have eyestrain or headaches for reasons unrelated to visual acuity. Good vision depends on much more than simply reading letters, as you'll see.

To test the acuity of your distance vision, stand twenty feet away from someone who is holding the book open to the Snellen chart shown on pages 5 through 8. Start reading each line of letters aloud with one eye covered, and have your friend turn the pages and check your answers. Then, switch to the other eye. Keep going down the chart until you reach the last line that you can comfortably read. The number next to that line tells you the acuity of your distance vision (20/20, 20/40 and so on). If your distance vision is not 20/20, you should see your eye doctor. You may need corrective lenses for distance (*see* text above for complete test instructions).

Distance Vision Test (Snellen Chart)

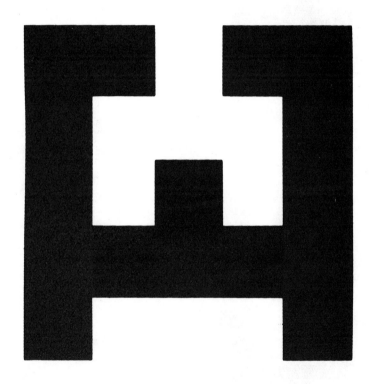

20 | 200

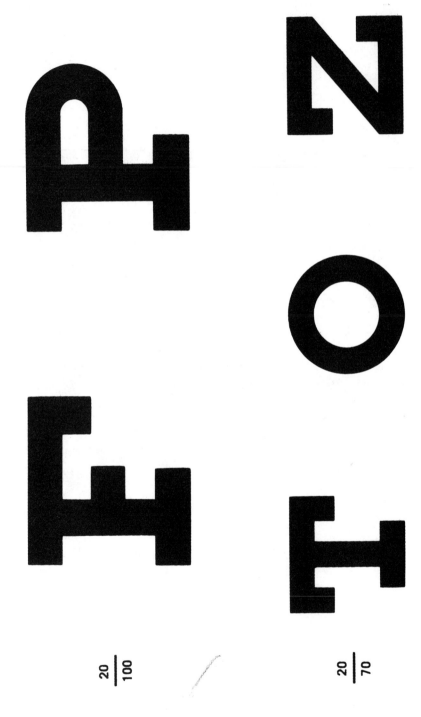

$\dfrac{20}{100}$ $\dfrac{20}{70}$

D E P L

D F C E P

P Z C F D E

D N P Z O F E F

20/50

20/40

20/30

20/25

C E T O P F E D

T C D O F E L

O E C T L P D F

D A F T C L O Z E P

$\frac{20}{20}$

$\frac{20}{15}$

$\frac{20}{13}$

$\frac{20}{10}$

**Near Vision Test
(Reduced Snellen Chart)**

E
NZ
Y L S
U F V P
N S T R F
R C L C T B
H T V P F R U

To test the acuity of your near vision, hold the book sixteen inches from your eyes, cover one eye, and see how far down the chart you can comfortably read. Now try the other eye. If you can read the bottom line of the chart from sixteen inches away, you have normal near vision. If you can't, you should see your eye doctor. You may need corrective lenses for reading.

Legally Blind?

Often I have patients coming in telling me that they are "legally blind." Well, let's get this one straight before running scared. According to the official government requirements, a person is legally blind when his or her vision is 20/200 or worse *with best correction.* It actually doesn't matter how poor your vision is *without* glasses or contact lenses as long as it is correctable to better than 20/200 *with* them. So, most of you are still well within those guidelines, and we hope to keep you there!

Test Your Near-Vision Acuity

Near vision is tested separately from distance vision. To test your near vision, you can use the illustration above, a reduced Snellen chart. Hold the book sixteen inches away from your eyes, cover one eye at a time, and start reading the chart. People with normal near-vision acuity can read the last line of the reduced Snellen chart. If you have trouble with that line, you may need reading glasses now or in the near future.

WHAT IS ASTIGMATISM?

One of the most common words heard around optometrists' offices is the one least understood. Yes, it's *astigmatism* (a-STIG-ma-tism).

First, we'll need to teach you some basic anatomy. The first surface that light strikes on its way through your eye is the cornea—the clear dome in the front of the eye that you saw earlier with your mirror. After it passes through the cornea, the next solid structure it encounters is the eye's *lens*, which changes shape to focus an image on the back of the eye (see *How You Focus Your Eyes*, page 18). Theoretically, the surface of the cornea should be almost spherical in shape, like the surface of a ball, so that when light passes through it, it can be focused at a single point. However, nature isn't always perfect, and the cornea is often "warped" so that it more closely resembles a barrel than a ball. The lens, too, can be irregular in shape. These distortions can be significant enough so that the light that passes through the cornea and lens in the vertical orientation will focus at a different spot from the light that passes through in the horizontal orientation. Now you have two points of focus with a blur between them. If the difference between these two points of focus is great enough, the eye will strain trying to decide which point of focus it should use. You might then develop occasional blurring of vision, fatigue or possibly headaches.

Astigmatism in small amounts is very common and not of great concern. But, about twenty-three million Americans have a significant amount of astigmatism, which requires correction. Glasses correct astigmatism by having curvatures that compensate for the curvature of the eye. This is a simple optical correction, and the glasses will not change the amount of astigmatism; i.e., they won't "cure" the problem. It is rare that exercises can help this type of problem since the cause is usually the physical distortion of the cornea.

Do You Have Astigmatism?

Testing yourself for astigmatism is going to be a bit tricky. This test will give you a general impression of astigmatism, but only a complete exam will be able to tell for sure.

Hold a magnifying glass in front of one eye while you look at the letters in the illustration on page 11 at your usual reading distance. If you have some astigmatism, the stripes in one or two of the letters will appear to be darker than those in the others. The direction of your astigmatism will determine which letters will stand out. If you have no appreciable amount of astigmatism, all the striped letters will look the same.

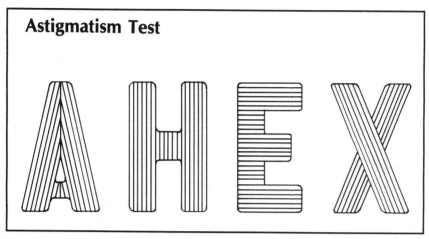

Astigmatism Test

To test yourself for astigmatism, cover one eye and hold a magnifying glass in front of the eye you are testing. Look at the striped letters at your usual reading distance. If some of them appear darker than others, you may have astigmatism and should see your eye doctor (*see* text on page 10 for complete test instructions).

So now you know that astigmatism is not an "eyestrain" in the usual sense of muscle strain, but it can certainly *cause* eyestrain as you try to compensate for it. If the letters in the illustration above show significant differences when you look at them, you should have an examination to see if there is enough astigmatism to create a problem with your vision.

YOUR PERIPHERAL (SIDE) VISION

Right now you're reading the words on this page with (I hope) both eyes. They are pointed down here, and all you are really aware of is the page you see. But if someone were to sneak up behind you and then slowly come around to your side, you'd probably see him move and know he was there (assuming he didn't tip you off by knocking over a chair). But how could you see someone off to your side if your eyes are looking down here? You were using your *peripheral*, or side, vision, which accounts for a large percentage of your whole *visual field*, which is all of what you can see at one time without turning your eyes. A normal visual field is about 170 degrees around, although certain conditions can narrow it. (In fact, another definition of "legally blind" is a visual field of less than twenty degrees.)

About half of the inside of your eye is lined by the *retina* (RET-nah), which is a light-sensitive membrane. When you look straight at an object, you line up that object with the *macula* (MAC-yoo-lah), a tiny, a one-square-millimeter area of the retina that gives you the sharpest vision (*see* illustration, page 36). So there's a whole lot of retina that isn't completely "tuned in" to where you're looking. But, when a person comes up beside you, he moves enough to alert the rest of your retina that something is there.

Peripheral vision is very important in driving a car, for example, because you use it to catch glimpses of cars on either side of you without actually turning your head or eyes completely around.

Test Your Peripheral Vision

To test your own peripheral vision, you'll need another person. Sit facing your friend about two feet apart at about the same eye level (*see* illustration, page 13). You'll need to use an object that can can be held at a slight distance from your hand, such as the eraser on a pencil. Have your friend cover one eye and you cover the opposite one (for example, her right, your left). Now extend the eraser all the way to the right as far as you can reach. Both of you must keep looking directly at each other's eye without moving. Slowly bring the eraser in toward yourself and the other person, but keep it on an imaginary line midway between you and your friend—you'll need to bend your elbow to do this. You should each see the eraser come into view out of the "corner" of your eye at about the same time. Be sure it's the eraser you see and not the pencil. If one person sees it *much* sooner than the other—when it is several inches farther away—the one who sees it last might have decreased peripheral vision and should get it checked more thoroughly. (A difference of six inches may be significant.)

Now do the exercise again, but this time come in from the left, and then again from the top and from the bottom, keeping one eye covered and looking straight ahead. Each time, the eraser should be seen at about the same time by both people. Then do your other eye, remembering to have your partner switch eyes also.

The test you've done is a gross estimate that will only pick up very significant problems. More accurate testing would need to be done to find more subtle defects in the visual field.

Peripheral Vision Test

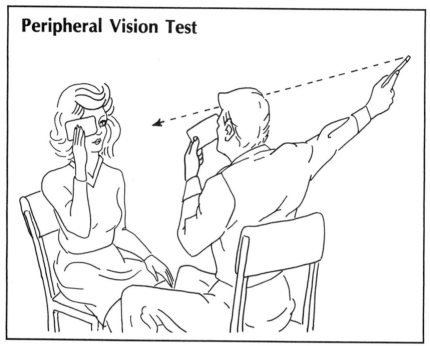

To test your peripheral vision, have a friend sit opposite you about two feet away. You cover your left eye while your friend covers her right eye. Hold a pencil, eraser end up, at arm's length out to your right side, and then slowly bring it in toward you and your friend, keeping it on an imaginary midline between the two of you. You should both see the eraser appear out of the "corner" of one eye at about the same time. Now cover the other eye and come in with the eraser from the opposite side. Also try coming in with the eraser from the top and from the bottom as you keep looking straight ahead with one eye covered. Each time, the eraser should be seen at about the same time by both people. If it isn't, the person who sees it last may have a problem with his or her peripheral vision and should have it checked more thoroughly by a doctor (*see* text on page 12 for complete test instructions).

It doesn't really take much to check out your eyes. Get to know them. Look at your eyelashes, eyebrows, upper and lower eyelids and your eyeballs. Get an idea of how your eyes feel in relation to how *you* feel. You'd be surprised at how your eyes tell others how you are feeling. Your eyes are truly a mirror to the soul.

Eye Openers

• Sight accounts for 90 to 95 percent of all sensory perceptions.

• On a clear night when there is no moon, a person sitting on a mountain peak can see a match struck fifty miles away.

• It is impossible to sneeze and keep your eyes open at the same time.

• In dim light, your peripheral vision is actually better than your central vision. Next time you want to look at a star, try focusing on a point adjacent to it instead of looking straight at it. You'll see the star better that way.

CHAPTER 2

Beyond Basics— More Eye Tests You Can Do

These simple tests don't require much equipment and are fun to do. You'll probably be trying some things you've never done before so don't worry if you don't succeed with every test on the first try.

SEEING THE INSIDE OF YOUR EYE

The retina—that's the light-sensitive membrane that lines the back of your eye—receives much of its blood supply from blood vessels that enter it from behind and then come to lie on its front surface. Light entering your eye must go past these vessels, and they therefore cast shadows on the retina. However, since these vessels are in the same place all the time, they cast shadows on the same areas of the retina all the time; your eyes have adapted to these shadows so that they are not visible to you under normal cirumstances.

Branching Blood Vessels

All you have to do to see these shadows is to completely darken the room and, while you're looking straight ahead, shine a bright flashlight into your eye from the side. Now move the flashlight back and forth next to your eye. You should see what

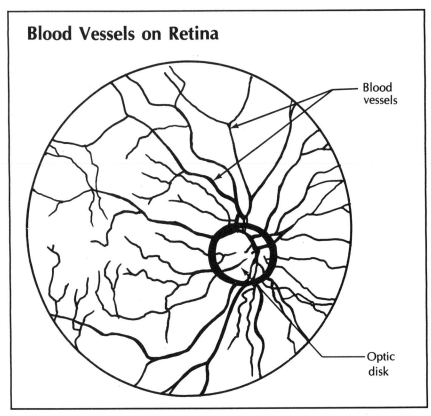

Blood Vessels on Retina

Blood vessels

Optic disk

The blood vessels on the retina form a branching pattern, which can be seen by shining a flashlight into your eye from the side in a darkened room. The optic disk is an area of the retina where the optic nerve leaves the eye, heading for the brain (see *The Eye-Brain Connection*, page 38 for more about the optic nerve).

look like large branches of a tree with no leaves. You are actually seeing the branching pattern of the blood vessels inside your eye (*see* illustration above).

Spots in Front of Your Eyes?

People often talk of seeing small dark spots in front of their eyes, which seem to move as they move their eyes. These spots may look like dots, squiggles, strands or hundreds of different shapes and are usually normal. They exist because, before birth, your eye develops by having blood vessels grow through the center of it. During the last three months of fetal life, these vessels dissolve, but sometimes they don't disappear completely. So what you are seeing are small strands of old blood vessels that are floating in the central gel part of your eye. They're actually called *floaters*. Floaters can also occur when protein fibers from the gel in your eye clump together. You may notice that these will be more obvious when you are looking at bright areas, such as blank walls or the white pages of a book, or you may even see them when your eyes are closed, especially if you're lying in the sun.

These floaters are harmless and there is no practical treatment for them. One word of caution, however: **If you suddenly become aware of hundreds of these floaters that appear all of a sudden, or if they are associated with flashes of light in your vision, it's advisable to check with an eye doctor to make sure there is nothing seriously wrong.**

The Electric Retina

Another fun test to do is to just cover your eyes gently with the palms of your hands. After a few seconds you may notice a few flashes of light. These dim flashes represent a natural electrical discharge of your retina. The retina is always in a state of electrical excitability, and even in complete darkness it can fire impulses of light.

Stimulating the Retina

This next test works better in a dark room, but you can also try it in normal light. Look as far to the left as you can and gently press your finger against your upper right eyelid just at the outer junction where your lids meet. You'll see a flash of light right near where you're looking. Now look as far to the right as you can and press your finger against your upper left eyelid; you should see the same flash. You'll also be able to see it with your eyes closed.

The flash is called a *pressure phosphene* (FAHS-feen), and it's produced when pressure is applied to the retina because any stimulus to the retina registers as light stimulation. (Pressure phosphenes occur when any part of the retina is stimulated, but you can see them best when you touch the outer corners of your eyes.) Did you ever wonder how people see "stars" when they get hit in the eye? Now you know!

HOW YOU FOCUS YOUR EYES

You may never have realized that your eye changes focus. Focusing happens so quickly and with such little effort in young people that it's hardly noticeable. As the process gets slower and more difficult with age, though, it becomes more obvious.

You've probably heard that the eye is like a camera. Well, it's not quite as simple as that. True, a camera does change focus, but it does so by moving a lens back and forth to clear the image. Your eye also has a lens, but the eye's lens doesn't move back and forth; instead, it *changes shape* to focus an image. This process of changing shape is called *accommodation*, although the term is most often used to describe the change from distance to near vision.

The eye's lens is controlled by a muscle. When the muscle is relaxed, the lens is biconvex in shape, resembling the shape of a lentil bean (which is what "lens" means in Latin). In this shape, the lens is focused for distance vision. When you want to see something close up—less than twenty feet away—the muscle contracts, causing a rounding of the lens.

What's So Special About Twenty Feet?

Ever wonder what's so special about twenty feet? At twenty feet or more from your eyes, the lens does not have to accommodate; it stays relaxed (biconvex). To understand the reason for this we'll need to do some lightweight physics. Light from any source radiates in all different directions, like a sparkler (*see* illustration, page 19). The light rays actually keep diverging from each other forever. But, when the object is twenty feet or more from the eye, the light rays from it strike the eye nearly parallel to each other. The lens can focus these parallel rays in its relaxed shape. For this reason, twenty feet is used as the standard for measuring distance vision—which is vision that doesn't require the lens to accommodate.

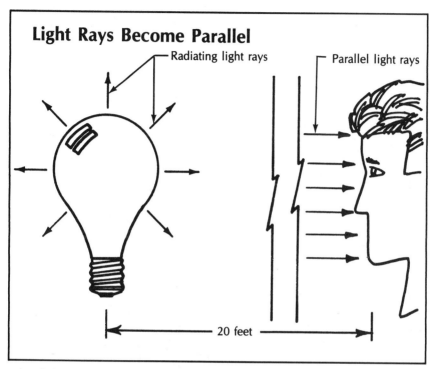

Light Rays Become Parallel

Radiating light rays

Parallel light rays

20 feet

When light rays are twenty feet or more away from the eye, they strike the eye nearly parallel to each other. When the light rays are parallel, the eye's lens does not have to accommodate in order to focus them on the retina. This is the reason for using twenty feet as a standard in measuring distance, as opposed to near, vision.

Test Your Focusing Ability

Here's how to test your focusing ability:

1. Take an index card and cut a circle an inch in diameter in the middle of it. Print some small letters around the hole (*see* illustration page 20).

2. Attach some newspaper headlines to a wall that is at least twenty feet away.

3. Hold the card at your usual reading distance, cover one eye, and line up the letters on the wall through the hole.

4. Notice as you look at those letters *through* the hole that the small letters *around* the hole are very blurred. That's because your eyes are focused for distance vision.

5. Look at the letters around the hole and notice that the letters on the wall are now blurred. That's because your eyes are

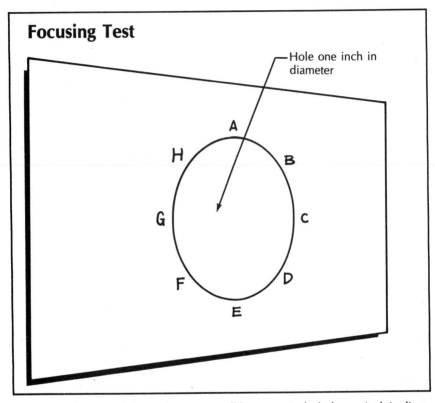

Focusing Test

Hole one inch in diameter

A
H
B
G
C
F
D
E

To test your focusing ability, print some small letters around a hole one inch in diameter in the center of a three-by-five-inch card. Attach some large letters (such as newspaper headlines) to a wall at least twenty feet away. When you're looking at the large letters on the wall, you'll notice that the small letters around the hole are blurred. When you're looking at the small letters around the hole, you'll notice that the large letters on the wall are blurred. This phenomenon occurs because your eyes are changing focus for near and distance vision (*see* text on page 20 for complete test instructions).

focused for near vision. You just changed the focus of your eyes—good work.

6. Go back to the large letters on the wall. Are they clear again?

This phenomenon occurs so constantly that you may never notice it unless you make yourself become aware of it.

The ability to focus for near and distance vision and back again is related to your age. Younger folks have a greater ability to focus. This relationship is so well established that a standard is used to correlate age and focusing ability (*see* box, page 21).

How Age Affects Accommodation

Age in Years	Distance at Which Vision Blurs in Inches
10	3.0
15	3.5
20	4.0
25	4.5
30	6.0
35	8.0
40	9.0
45	11.0
50	16.0
55	23.0
60	40.0
65	80.0

This table shows maximum focusing ability, or accommodation. Most people can maintain this amount of accommodation for a short time. For reading and other activities requiring near vision, only one-half of our maximum ability can comfortably be used. To read the chart for "comfortable reading distance," double the distance for your age group. Now you know why after the age of forty our arms don't seem long enough to maintain clear focus on reading material. That's about when the "bifocal age" occurs (see *Presbyopia—Or, Your Short Arms*, page 81).

Look at the small letters around the hole in your card again, and slowly bring them closer toward you. (If you wear glasses, keep them on.) When they first begin to blur, stop. Have a friend measure how far the card is away from your eyes. If you need more distance for near vision than that in the table on page 21 (in other words, if things look blurry when they're close to your eyes), it means that your ability to focus is not as good as that of most people your age. Only a complete vision examination can tell if that should be a concern for you.

The time it takes to change focus is also important. It should take only a half a second to focus from far to near, and no more than one second to focus from near to far. If it takes you longer than this, your eyes are probably struggling to focus and it's time for an eye exam. Focusing ability can often be improved with exercises. I'll talk more about that in chapter 9.

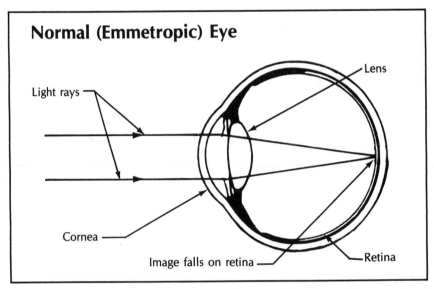

Normal (Emmetropic) Eye

Lens

Light rays

Cornea

Image falls on retina

Retina

In the normal eye, an image falls exactly on the retina. The shape of the eyeball and cornea are normal, and the eye's lens has normal flexibility and focusing ability.

NEARSIGHTED OR FARSIGHTED?

First, let's try to get these terms straightened out. *Near-sightedness*, also called *myopia* (my-OH-pee-ah), means having good near vision but poor distance vision. For the myopic person, a distant image (any image at least twenty feet away, so that the eye's lens is as relaxed as it can be) falls *in front of* the retina and looks blurred (*see* illustration, page 23). Nearsightedness results when an eye is too long, when the cornea is too steeply curved, when the eye's lens is unable to relax enough to provide accurate distance vision or from some combination of these and other factors.

Farsightedness, also called *hyperopia* (hy-per-OH-pee-ah), is not exactly the opposite of myopia. For the hyperopic person, an object that is twenty feet or more away (so that the lens is relaxed) is focused *in back of* the retina, and it looks blurred (*see* illustration, page 23). Farsightedness results when an eye is too short or the cornea too flat or from some combination of these and other factors.

Myopia, hyperopia and astigmatism are all known as *refractive errors* because they cause distortions in the way light is *refracted*—deflected from a straight path—as it goes through the

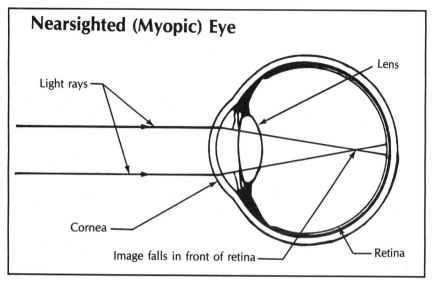

Nearsighted (Myopic) Eye

Light rays

Lens

Cornea

Image falls in front of retina

Retina

In the nearsighted eye, the image falls in front of the retina when the lens is in its relaxed state, viewing an object that is at least twenty feet away. The image is blurred. Nearsightedness can be caused by an eye that is too long, a cornea that is too steep, a lens that cannot relax enough to focus distant images or by a combination of these and other factors.

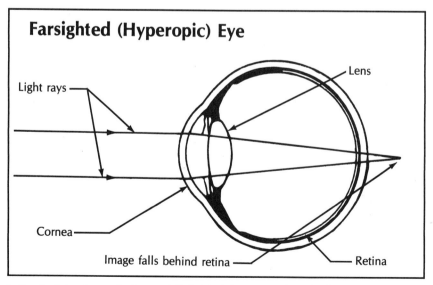

Farsighted (Hyperopic) Eye

Light rays

Lens

Cornea

Image falls behind retina

Retina

In the farsighted eye, the image falls behind the retina when the lens is in its relaxed state, viewing an object that is at least twenty feet away. The image is blurred. Farsightedness can be caused by an eye that is too short, a cornea that is too flat or by a combination of these and other factors.

eye. The condition of the optically normal eye has a name too; it's called *emmetropia* (em-e-TROH-pee-ah).

Pinhole Tests

You now know what 20/20 vision means and can use the eye chart to measure it. There are also some other ways to tell whether or not your eyesight is as accurate as it should be.

To try these tests for near- and farsightedness, you'll need a small piece of paper with a tiny pinhole in it. Close one eye and look at some distant object (at least twenty feet away). Hold the pinhole up in front of your eye (no glasses now) and notice if the object you were looking at got any clearer. If the object cleared up, you are probably nearsighted. (Nearsighted people get the same effect from squinting.) If you're farsighted, the object probably just got dimmer. A similar test can be done with the same equipment. Hold the pinhole so it is about four inches in front of your eye. Look at that distant object (at least twenty feet away) through the hole and move the paper from side to side. The object will appear to move also. If the object moves in the same direction as the paper, you're myopic. If it moves the opposite way, you're hyperopic. Seems like a fairly simple test, doesn't it? It will give you a pretty fair idea if your eyesight is as sharp as it should be, although it doesn't replace a complete vision examination.

TWO EYES, ONE PICTURE

One of the most fascinating abilities of the visual system is to take images from two eyes and put them together into just one picture. You don't normally see two images, so the idea might sound strange, but double vision can occur and is one of the most dangerous manifestations of vision problems. Imagine seeing two cars coming at you as you drive down the road!

Here's how the brain keeps us from going off the road. Let's assume that you have two eyes and they are both working about equally well. As you look at just one object, each eye receives an image of that object. Both of these images are transmitted back to your brain, but they are then "fused" together by the brain into one image. In order for that to happen, both eyes must be pointed in the same direction, and the images have to be approximately equal in size and clarity.

Now, if one eye does not aim at the same spot as the other, each eye will be "looking" at a different object, and the two images won't match up. When the images are transmitted back to your brain, they will stimulate two different groups of brain cells, and you will experience two images: You will see double. After a short time, your brain will decide to "turn off," or suppress, the picture from the eye that is pointed in the wrong direction so that you can see one image again. This suppression is necessary for our visual survival, but it is not the way we were made to see. A complete eye examination is necessary to uncover a double vision problem and to correct it.

Seeing Double

Grab two of your favorite pencils and hold one of them in front of your nose — about six inches away. Hold the other extended at arm's length in line with your nose and the other pencil. Now look at the closer pencil, but be aware of the further one. If both eyes are working together properly, you should see two pencils at the extended point but only one where you are looking at near. You might have to jiggle the extended one a bit to achieve this effect. Now, keep the pencils where they are, but look at the extended pencil. As you do, you should notice that the closer pencil is doubled. You won't see this doubling if both eyes aren't working together properly.

This test should illustrate that you are really seeing double all the time! You use this doubling of the visual field to help maintain balance and in other visual activities. So, having two eyes is a definite advantage and you should be sure that they are working together.

PUPIL SIZE

As you know from reading chapter 1, the pupil is just a hole in the iris that lets light get through to the retina. When the light is bright, the pupils get smaller to cut down on the amount of light entering the eyes; when you're in the dark, your pupils get larger to catch as much light as possible.

The pupil, however, does react to more than just light. In fact, the pupil (really the iris) is in constant motion, getting bigger and smaller for a number of reasons.

Both pupils should always be about the same size (25 percent of the population has *slightly* unequal pupils) and both react at the same time to any stimulus. If you notice any differences between your two pupils, consult your optometrist or ophthalmologist.

Tickle Test

Have a friend tickle your ear (or anything that is ticklish) while you're looking at your pupils in the mirror. If you can stand the excitement, you'll notice that your pupils will dilate (enlarge) slightly when you feel the goose bumps. They also dilate when looking at pleasing pictures, seeing food when you're hungry, solving easy math problems and opening your eyes every time after a blink.

Blink Test

Use your pinhole in a piece of paper again and hold it about an inch in front of one eye. Cover the other eye and look at a bright surface. As you blink you'll see the size of the hole change (it gets larger, then smaller). What is actually changing is the size of your pupil.

HOW YOUR EYES MOVE

It has been said that vision is really a *motor function*—that is, a function that is performed by moving musles. In fact, eye movement is essential to vision. Our eyes are controlled by two sets of six eye muscles, one set for each eye (*see* illustration, page 27). These muscles are attached to the outer coat of the eye on one end and to bones within the skull at the other. You should be aware that your eyes are in motion all the time, and it's important that they move smoothly and with control.

Good eye movements involve more than just strong eye muscles. The eye muscles involved with these types of movements are a hundred times as strong as they need to be to move an eyeball. What is important, however, is muscle *coordination*, which starts in your brain, not in your eyes.

Rotation Test

Watching your own eyes move isn't too easy to do so you'll need a friend. Grab a pencil and have your friend watch the tip

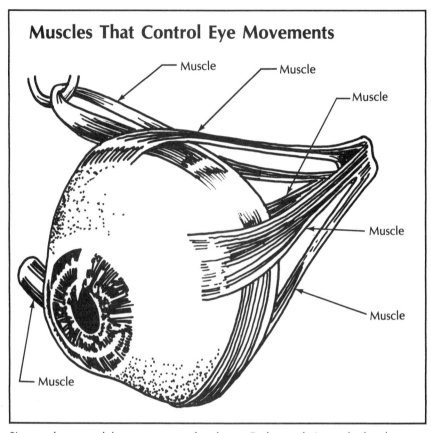

Muscles That Control Eye Movements

Muscle

Muscle

Muscle

Muscle

Muscle

Muscle

Six muscles control the movements of each eye. Each muscle is attached to the outer coat of the eye on one end and to bones in the skull at the other end. Each is capable of pulling the eye in a slightly different direction.

of it as you rotate it in front of his or her eyes (*see* illustration, page 28). Stay at least a foot away and move the pencil slowly in a large circle. Watch your friend's eyes—no head movements allowed—as he follows the pencil tip; the movements should be smooth and continuous. If you notice any jerky eye movements, or if your friend seems to lose sight of the pencil, then his or her eye control isn't what it should be. Now switch places and have someone watch *your* eyes.

Eye Shifts

There's another kind of eye movement that's also important. While you read, your eyes make small "jumping" motions across

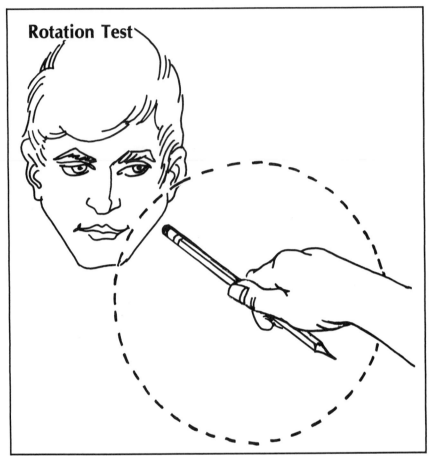

Rotation Test

To see if someone has smooth eye movements, rotate a pencil in a large circle at least a foot away from the person's eyes. Have the person watch the pencil without moving his or her head. The movements should be smooth and continuous (*see* text on page 26 for complete test instructions).

the page. You may be able to see these if you look at someone's eyes as the person reads. Most readers average about eleven jumps per line. This type of jumping or shifting movement is called a *saccade* (sa-KAYD).

Hold up one finger of each hand about two feet apart in front of your friend. Ask your friend to look at one finger and then the other without making any head movements. As his eyes shift from one finger to the other, notice that his eyes may jump one, two or even three times until they land directly on the target. This movement is similar to eye movements made during reading. The fewer jumps per line required to land on the target, the better. Making this type of movement smoothly and continuously is essential for reading efficiency and comprehension.

Convergence Test

Another kind of movement is called *convergence*, which means "coming together." When you look at a distant object, your eyes aim straight ahead. If you now look at a closer object, your eyes will turn in toward each other (converge). This is normal.

Have a friend look at the tip of your finger as you slowly move it toward her nose from about twenty inches away. Her eyes should follow it almost all the way to the tip of her nose. If one eye stops turning in, or if your friend sees double while your finger is still more than four inches away, an eye exam is in order. (At four inches or closer, seeing double is normal.)

Convergence is essential for efficient reading, and without effortless convergence, close work will be difficult and tiring.

Drifting Eyes

Most people's eyes have a tendency to drift toward or away from what they are looking at. This tendency is usually not apparent in normal visual situations, so you'll have to try this test to see if someone has drifting eyes:

1. Have a friend focus on the tip of your finger at about twelve inches from his eyes while you cover one of his eyes with your hand.

2. Uncover your friend's eye. If the eye moves in toward the nose after it is uncovered, then it has drifted outward while covered. If it moves away from the nose after being uncovered, you'll know it has drifted inward while it was covered.

3. Try quickly alternating the cover from eye to eye. Is there any movement of the eye that is covered and then uncovered?

If there is no eye movement, then your friend has good balance of his eye muscles. Now switch places and have your friend test you. You may have to test several people to see both kinds of drifting.

This tendency of the eyes to drift outward or inward has to be overcome for the eyes to converge efficiently, so if your eyes tend to turn *out* quite a lot, it may be difficult to converge them for any length of time, as you have to do while reading. If the tendency is to turn *in*, then they will have to learn to relax the convergence while doing close work. This drifting tendency is not always an easy task for the visual system to accomplish.

YOUR DOMINANT EYE

Close one eye. OK—which eye did you close? In everyday seeing, do you feel that one eye does see just a little better than the other one? Most of us have one eye that "leads" over the other; it is called the dominant eye and it may or may not be a significant factor in your seeing ability.

If it is true that two eyes are better than one, then why should one be dominant? First of all, there are going to be times when you need only one eye—for instance, in aligning things or aiming at an object with a camera or telescope. In these cases you'll find yourself closing one eye to get an exact alignment. The brain normally chooses the better eye for the job.

Many people have one eye that is very different from its mate. One eye may be farsighted and the other nearsighted, or astigmatism may occur in just one eye. In any case, the eye that sees the most clearly while doing the least amount of work will be the one chosen to do the seeing. The eye you choose may not always be the same one in every situation. A nearsighted eye can read up close more easily than a farsighted eye, but the farsighted one can pick out a distant street sign more easily.

Considerable research has been done to try to determine the significance of dominant eyes, hands and feet. Some authorities say that if all three are the same (for example, if a child is right-eyed, right-handed and right-footed), the dominance is complete, allowing for normal development of perception. If the dominance is mixed, say these researchers, there is confusion within the brain, and the child has difficulty learning to distinguish between left and right. Some experts believe that mixed dominance is a significant factor in *dyslexia*—difficulty learning to read—and other learning disabilities.

However, there is an equal amount of evidence that refutes these findings and says that mixed dominance is not necessarily a problem. No evidence has yet convinced me of the necessity for complete dominance, although I do believe it is important for a child to develop good left-right discrimination (see *Sequence of Visual-Motor Development*, page 47).

Eye dominance is an intriguing area to study, and much information is available on the subject. The normal dominance of one eye over the other is not likely to cause you any visual problems. However, if you notice a difference in the vision of one eye versus the other, a thorough examination is indicated.

Dominance Test

To test your dominant eye you'll need your three-by-five-inch card with the one-inch hole in the middle of it.

1. Hold the card with both hands at arm's length and *keep both eyes open.* Use any small target at a far distance and line up the target in the hole.

2. Close your right eye while still holding the card steady. If the target disappears, then you were using your right eye to align it and your right eye is dominant. If you closed your right eye and you still saw the target, then you were using your left eye to align it, and your left eye is dominant.

DEPTH PERCEPTION

There are really two ways to perceive depth. "True" depth comes only when a person can use both eyes together. This perception is called *stereopsis* (ster-ee-AHP-sis).

Stereopsis occurs when two eyes point at one object, each from a slightly different angle. This angle serves to "bring out" the true depth of the object so that you can tell exactly how far away it is and whether it is in front of or behind a similar object near it. Stereopsis has to do with your visual perception and does not have to be learned.

The second kind of depth perception is called *perspective.* When you see things in perspective, you're using clues to depth that are not part of your perception, but rather must be learned by the thinking part of your brain.

For instance, if you hold a quarter up to the moon, close to your eye, you can block out the moon completely. A small child might rely only on his visual perception here and think the quarter was actually larger than the moon. You and I know — because we've learned it — that the moon is much bigger than the quarter, so we correctly judge that the quarter only appears bigger because it is very near to us and the moon is very far away.

Let's try another example. You are driving down a highway and notice that a telephone pole near your car appears larger than the poles further down the road. They are actually the same size, but your perception makes the closer pole look bigger. Here again, without your acquired knowledge that the poles are very likely to be the same size, you might be misled by your visual perception. But, your knowledge that the poles are the same size allows you to perceive that the "smaller" ones are the more distant, and the "larger" ones are simply closer.

Where's the Pencil?

Did you ever notice how everything flattens out when you close one eye? Maybe not, but try it. What you're doing is eliminating your stereoscopic visual cues. Just look around the room and try to forget that you know what's closer and what's farther away — in other words, eliminate your learned cues too. It may take a minute or two to accomplish this "forgetting." While your eye is still covered, have someone hold a pencil about two feet in front of you. Take your forefinger and try to touch the pencil tip as you approach it from one side. Chances are that you'll miss it by a little.

True depth perception is best with two good eyes. Are your eyes working well together?

BLIND SPOTS

When I was in grade school, someone told me that everyone had a blind spot in their eyes. I looked and looked, but I could always see everything I looked at. I was convinced that there wasn't really a blind spot in *my* eye. I probably would not believe it today if I hadn't seen it for myself.

The back of the inside of your eye is covered with the retina, which receives light and transmits nerve impulses to the brain. The cells in the retina are connected to nerve fibers that lead to your brain. These fibers collectively make up the *optic nerve.* The area where the optic nerve leaves the retina heading for the brain is not covered with retinal cells, but is solely the exit for nerve fibers. Since it has no cells to receive light, no perception occurs in this area; it is actually blind. This area is called the *optic disk* (*see* illustration, page 16 and page 36).

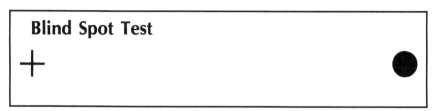

To find the blind spot in your right eye, cover your left eye and look at the plus sign on the left side of the page. Hold the book about six inches from your eyes, and then slowly move it back until it is about twelve inches from your eyes. When the book is about twelve inches from you, the black dot on the right side of the page should disappear. To find the blind spot in your left eye, cover your right eye and look at the large dot on the right side of the page. Hold the book about six inches from your eyes, and then move it back until it is about twelve inches away. The plus sign should disappear when the book is about twelve inches away from you (*see* text below for complete test instructions).

Blind Spot Test

There is one blind spot in each eye so you may test either eye first.

1. Look at the illustration above. There is a plus sign on the left side of the page and a large dot on the right side.

2. Look at the plus sign if you're testing your right eye; if you're testing the left eye, you'll look at the dot (no, I didn't say that backwards!). Cover the eye that is not being tested.

3. Hold the book six inches from your eyes, remembering to keep the eye you're not testing covered. Now, slowly move the book back to about twelve inches from your face.

4. Look directly at the plus sign with your right eye; the dot on the right side of the page will disappear from the corner of your vision at about twelve inches from your eyes. You may have to move back and forth or left and right a bit to get this effect because the blind spot is not very big. Remember to keep the uncovered eye still and directed straight ahead.

5. Try the other eye next.

OK, so you have found this blind spot in each eye. Why don't you normally see any empty space in that area? Well, if you remember, you have two eyes, right? Each one has a visual field or area of visual perception. The fields of your two eyes overlap quite a bit, so there is a large area of *binocular*—two-eyed—vision. The blind spot in one eye is overlapped by a seeing portion of the other eye, so if both your eyes are open and functioning, you don't have any gaps in your visual field.

Blind spots are significant in the detection of eye diseases and other conditions, including brain tumors. For example, the eye disease *glaucoma* (glaw-KOH-mah), which involves an increase in pressure in the eye, will cause the blind spot to enlarge (see *Glaucoma*, page 89). Tracking the changes in the size of the blind spot can give a doctor information about the progression of a disease. If you ever perceive a blind area in your vision—other than the normal one I just showed you—be sure to have it checked immediately.

Eye Openers

• About 58 percent of Americans—about 143 million people—wear some form of vision correction.

• In countries where the metric system is used (all of Europe), 20/20 vision is called 6/6 vision, meaning you can see at six meters what the normal eye can see at six meters.

• The images of stars are always slightly displaced from their real position because light bends gradually when traveling through layers of air that have different densities.

CHAPTER 3
How Does Vision Work?

In learning about your eyes and how to take care of them, you should have some knowledge of how they're put together, and how they work in conjunction with the brain. As you read, refer to the illustrations on pages 36 and 37.

SEEING VERSUS VISION

In developmental optometry, *seeing* is given a different meaning from *vision*. "Seeing" describes what happens in the eye—the "eye-as-a-camera" part of how vision works. "Vision" adds what goes on once a signal from the eye reaches the brain. You might say that "seeing" is the ability to perceive what is there, while "vision" is the ability to get meaning out of what is there. It's something like the difference between "hearing" and "listening." Some of what vision entails is almost as automatic as seeing (such as jumping out of the way of a moving car), but some aspects of vision, such as how to fully interpret written language, have to be learned at the highest levels of the brain as they work with the eyes. So, let's see how seeing and vision work.

THE EYEBALL—
FORM FOLLOWS FUNCTION

The eyeball is basically that—a ball. Its diameter is roughly an inch, and it's about three inches in circumference. The part of

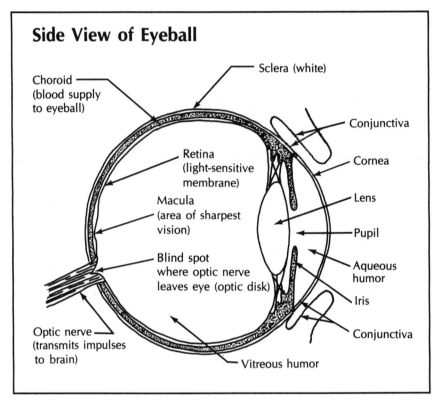

Side View of Eyeball

Choroid
(blood supply
to eyeball)

Sclera (white)

Conjunctiva

Retina
(light-sensitive
membrane)

Cornea

Macula
(area of sharpest
vision)

Lens

Pupil

Blind spot
where optic nerve
leaves eye (optic disk)

Aqueous
humor

Iris

Optic nerve
(transmits impulses
to brain)

Conjunctiva

Vitreous humor

The eye is a ball approximately one inch in diameter and three inches in circumference. The conjunctiva is a thin, transparent membrane that lines the upper and lower eyelids and also covers the "white" of the eye. The "white" of the eye is made of tough fibers that form the outermost layer of the eyeball; it's called the sclera. The cornea is a clear portion of the sclera, and it covers the central part of the eyeball (roughly corresponding to the area of the iris) the way glass or plastic covers the face of a watch. The choroid, a layer just inside the sclera, contains blood vessels that supply the inner eyeball. The lens of the eye changes shape to focus images on the retina, which is a light-sensitive membrane lining the back of the eye. The iris is a colored membrane between the lens and the cornea; it contracts and dilates, regulating the size of the pupil and the amount of light that enters the eye. The part of the eye in front of the lens is filled with a watery substance called aqueous fluid. The part of the eye in back of the lens is filled with a gel known as vitreous humor. The optic nerve transmits impulses from the retina to the brain. The part of the retina where the optic nerve is located is a blind area because it has no light-sensitive cells. This area is also called the optic disk. The macula is the part of the retina with the greatest density of light-sensitive cells, making it the area of sharpest vision.

How Eyes and Brain Connect

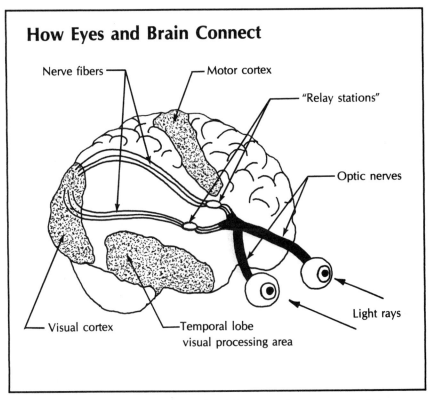

When light rays strike the rods and cones of the retina, they convert the light energy to nerve energy—a visual impulse. Visual impulses travel from the eye to the brain at 423 miles per hour. It is believed that they travel first to a pair of "relay stations" in the middle of the brain, where they are combined with information from other sensory organs (from the ears, for example). Visual impulses then travel to the visual cortex at the back of the brain, where visual information is interpreted. Further visual processing is done in the temporal lobe processing area. After the vision centers of the brain have interpreted the information from the eyes, they relay signals to other parts of the brain, such as the motor cortex, which controls movement.

the eye that is visible to the world—between the eyelids—is actually only one-sixth of the eye's total surface area. The remaining five-sixths of the eyeball is hidden behind the eyelids.

The outer surface of the eye is divided into two parts: the *sclera*, the white part that you saw with your mirror in chapter 1, and the *cornea*, the transparent membrane in front, which you also saw when you first examined your eyes. The cornea, which is steeper in curvature than the sclera, may be difficult to see because it is transparent and because the colored iris is behind it. You can see the cornea most easily if you look at a friend's eye from the side.

The sclera is the outermost layer of the eyeball. It is made of tough fibers, which allow it to perform its function as the supporting structure for the contents of the eyeball. It has a white appearance because the fibers are light in color and because there are very few blood vessels in it.

Just inside the sclera and covering all of the same area is the *choroid* (KOH-royd), which is the main blood supply to the inner eyeball. And just inside the choroid is the retina.

In addition to the blood vessels of the choroid, there are also blood vessels that enter the eye through the *optic nerve* and lie on the front surface of the retina. They supply nutrition to the *retina* and other structures inside the eye.

These parts all seem to be very basic when you think of what an eye must do. The eye needs protection and support (provided by the sclera), a supply of blood (provided by the choroid and through the optic nerve) and a mechanism for seeing (provided by the retina).

As you look at an eye, the first thing you'll notice is the colored *iris*. If you look closely at the illustration on page 36, you'll see that the iris is actually in a closed space, which is known as a *chamber*. The iris is also surrounded by a watery fluid called the *aqueous* (AY-kwee-us) *humor* or *aqueous fluid*. ("Humor," by the way, doesn't have anything to do with being funny it's just the Latin word for "fluid.") Just behind the iris is the lens, which provides the focusing part of the vision process. The lens is transparent and can't really be seen from the outside unless special equipment is used. Behind it, and filling the main chamber within the eye, is the *vitreous* (VIT-ree-us) *humor*. The vitreous humor is more gel-like and less watery than the aqueous humor and helps in the support of the retina and other structures.

THE EYE-BRAIN CONNECTION

Let's start at the beginning. Light enters the eye by passing through the cornea, the aqueous humor and the pupil; is focused by the lens; and then goes through the vitreous humor and onto the retina. You may have heard that the retina is actually an extension of the brain. That's right! The nerve fibers from the retina go directly into the brain.

The light that strikes the retina first stimulates chemical changes in the light-sensitive cells of the retina, known as the *photoreceptors*. There are actually two kinds of photoreceptors: The *rods*, which are long, slender cells, respond to light or dark stimuli and are important to our night vision; the *cones*, which are cone-shaped, respond to color stimuli and therefore are also called *color receptors*. There are about seventeen times as many rods as there are cones—about 120 million rods and 7 million cones in the retina of each eye. These rods and cones interconnect and converge to form a network of about a million nerve fibers that make up the optic nerve.

When light strikes the rods and cones, they convert the light energy to nerve energy; we'll call this nerve energy a *visual impulse*. This impulse travels out of the eye into the brain via the optic nerve at a speed of 423 miles per hour. It first reaches the middle of the brain where, physiologists believe, a pair of "relay stations" combine the visual information it is carrying with other sensory information (*see* illustration, page 37). The impulse then travels to the very back part of the brain, the *visual cortex*. It is here that the brain interprets the shapes of objects and the spatial organization of a scene and recognizes visual patterns as belonging to a known object—for example, it recognizes that a flower is a flower. Further visual processing is done at the sides of the brain, known as the *temporal lobes*. Once the brain has interpreted vital information about something the eyes have "seen," it instantaneously transfers this information to many areas of the brain. For example, if the information is that a car is moving toward you, it is relayed to the *motor cortex*, which is the area that controls movement and enables you to get out of the way. It's located in a band that goes over the top of your head from just above one ear to just above the other ear.

So, vision is really the combination of the eyeball receiving the light and the brain interpreting the signals from the eye.

COLOR VISION

Before we can talk about color vision, we'll need to go over some basics about the nature of light.

In chapter 2, we talked about light rays coming from a source of light. These rays radiate from the light source like the waves formed in water when a rock hits its surface.

These waves travel in varying lengths, some shorter than others. The unit of length used to measure waves of light is the *nanometer* (nan-AHM-iter), which is one millionth of a milli-meter, or one billionth of a meter.

The range of light that we humans can see—called "visible light"—is light with a wavelength of between 400 and 700 nanometers (nm). (*Ultraviolet light* has a wavelength below four hundred nm, and the wavelength of *infrared light* is above seven hundred nm.)

Seeing Red

When white light bounces off a red apple, the apple absorbs all the light rays except for those with a wavelength of about 650 nm; these it reflects. We humans have learned to call this particular wavelength of reflected light "red." Each color that we can see has its own wavelength; blue is about 460 nm, green about 520 and yellow about 575 nm. When we perceive a colored object, what we see is that part of the light spectrum that is not absorbed by the object, but rather is reflected back to our eyes.

What Happens in the Retina and Brain

Strange as it may seem, we still don't know for sure what happens in the retina and brain to enable us to have color vision, but we do have some theories on the subject.

The *trichromatic* (try-kroh-MA-tik), meaning "three-color," theory says that there are three different types of cones in the retina. There are cones that respond to the color red, cones for blue and cones for green. When the cones receive a light stimulus, they send a message to the brain via nerve fibers. Color mixing is obtained by these cones firing in varying proportions, so that the color we perceive is a combination of the signals coming from the three types of cones. White, for example, is perceived when the red, blue and green cones fire together.

This is a pretty good working model for color vision, but it's probably not the whole story. There are probably receptors that transmit light stimuli of a particular wavelength from the retina to the brain, and other receptors that *inhibit* light stimuli of particular wavelengths. The color we actually perceive is probably a result of some "yes" receptors and some "no" receptors sending messages to the brain.

COLOR 'BLINDNESS'

For approximately 8 percent of men and 0.5 percent of women in this country (the numbers vary somewhat in different countries), something goes wrong. The color connection mechanism doesn't work properly, and they are sometimes called *color-blind.* Actually, the term "color-blind" is a misnomer, because nearly every person with this affliction has only a *deficiency,* not a total absence, in his or her ability to see a full range of colors.

People who are *color-deficient,* the term I prefer, are either missing a certain type of color cone in their retina, or their cones are deficient in their ability to process color signals.

When the red-receiving cones do not function properly or are absent, the person will have a defect in his or her perception of the color red. The technical term for "red blindness" is *protanopia* (proh-tan-OH-pee-ah). When the green-receiving cones are not functioning or are absent, there will be "green blindness," which is called *deuteranopia* (doo-ter-an-OH-pee-ah). Deficiencies in perceiving yellows and blues also occur, but they are extremely rare.

Although color deficiency can be acquired during a person's life because of certain diseases or as a side effect of certain drugs, it is more often genetically inherited and present from birth. Men are about fifteen times more likely to be color-deficient than are women because of the way in which color deficiency is inherited (see *The Eyes Before Birth,* page 50).

Color vision can be quickly and simply tested by your eye doctor. If it is determined that you have some form of color deficiency, fear not. Color problems do not affect visual acuity, and even the most color-deficient person can have 20/20 vision. If you want to be an electrical worker or a pilot, you probably need excellent color discrimination, but a color deficiency can be coped with in most occupations. Of course, it can be inconvenient. One of my patients said that she always knew when her color-deficient co-worker had had a disagreement with his wife; he would come to work in clothes that clashed.

YOUR TEARS AND THEIR FUNCTION

Your tears are very important for keeping your eyes working properly. They are normally secreted from the membrane that covers each of your eyes—the conjunctiva. But when it comes time for a sudden "burst" of tears, two glands, which are called the *lacrimal* (LAK-rim-al) *glands,* get called into action. These glands are located above each eye and get stimulated for a number of different reasons, some of which are: emotion (happy or sad), extremely bright light, physical contact or drying out of the cornea.

You may have noticed the tiny holes in your lower and upper eyelids near your nose. They are for drainage of the tears. (No, the tears aren't produced at those holes, as many people believe!) The tears get washed from the outer corners of your eyes and are collected at the inner corners of your eyes near your nose. The tiny holes drain the tears into your nasal sinuses, which is the reason some people go through a box of tissues blowing their noses when they cry. Tears pour onto your cheeks when the drainage areas have overflowed.

Your tears also maintain the clarity of your cornea. The cornea must be very clear so light can pass through easily. Tears help this by collecting oxygen from the air and maintaining the proper air-to-fluid balance in the cornea.

Let your tears do the work they are supposed to do. Don't mess up their action by using over-the-counter eye drops. You see, tears contain an *enzyme*—a protein that can cause changes in other substances without being changed itself—that fights off undesirable bacteria. If your eyes look red, there's a reason for it, and using commercial eye drops just covers up the symptoms.

EYELIDS

Eyelids are very important structures and should be treated kindly. They have quite a few different functions. First, and probably most importantly, they protect your eyes. Have you ever had a puff of air blown at your eye? You automatically blink. This reflex is the fastest one we have. When the nerves in your cornea get even the slightest disturbance, the signal goes to your eyelids to close.

Your eyelids are also responsible for the cleaning of your eyes. Since they're open most of the day, the eyes need to be cleaned fairly often—especially with the amount of dust and smog in our air today. The action of the eyelids is such that, when they close, the outer corners touch first, and they gradually continue closing to the inner corners to complete the blink.

Eye Openers

• Although the retina represents one-millionth of a person's total body weight, its nerve fibers represent 40 percent of the nerve fibers going to the brain.

• The brain and the visual system together represent only 2 percent of your body weight, but they use up about 25 percent of your nutritional intake.

• Your eyes take 50 percent of your energy to control 80 percent of your actions.

• Your eyes register thirty-six thousand visual messages each hour.

• The normal human eye can see the light of a candle that is fourteen miles away.

• The eye weighs one-sixtieth of what the heart weighs, but it uses one-third the amount of oxygen the heart uses.

• Your eyes can perceive about 150 different colors.

• Contrary to popular belief, most mammals are probably not color-blind (although a few nocturnal mammals, such as rats and hamsters, are). Dogs, for example, have recently been found to have two types of photoreceptors: One responds to the blue and violet end of the visual spectrum, and the other responds to reddish hues and can also dimly detect blues. Because the two receptors overlap in the blue spectrum, dogs have good color discrimination for blues, but they probably see greens, yellows, oranges and reds as one shade.

This creates a sweeping motion, and all the dust that collects in the tears gets washed toward your nose, where it can drain away.

When a blink cleans your eyes, it also spreads a new layer of tears on the eyeball to keep it moist and accessible to oxygen.

Another feature of your eyelids is that, when they close, the light reaching your eyes gets shut off, which gives your eyes a split second of rest. Since you normally blink about fourteen times a minute (more if you're talking), that can add up to a great deal of rest for your eyes. We always blink less often when we are reading or watching something intently, such as a TV, computer or movie screen. These are times you should be more aware of your blinking; notice when your eyes are getting tired or dry.

And finally, your eyelids are extremely important for one other feature: keeping the light out when you need an extra fifteen minutes of sleep in the morning.

CHAPTER 4
Children's Eyes

A young child may think that everyone sees the way he or she does. She may not realize that she's supposed to be able to see the leaves on a tree from across the street or the letters on a blackboard from the rear of a classroom. The child may not know she has a problem, but estimates are that one out of every twenty preschool children in the United States has a vision problem that will eventually lead to needless loss of sight or a severe learning disability. Eighty to 85 percent of our learning comes through our vision. It's our most important sense. Most vision problems can be corrected if detected early. So, as a parent, your job is to get in touch with your child and find out what is happening with her vision. *Your child's vision is your responsibility.*

This chapter will show you some techniques for testing your child's vision and for improving his visual perception. If you have any doubts about whether your child's vision is developing on schedule, I advise you to consult your pediatrician or eye-care professional. *Developmental optometrists* have a special interest in children's eyes and how they relate to the general maturation of the child.

Normal Vision Development

The structure of the eyeball closely resembles adult size by the age of three with some growth and refinement continuing into adulthood. However, there is much more to a child's vision than physical structure—the "more" is the difference between

What Is Vision Therapy?

Some optometrists specialize in what's known as *vision therapy*. Back in the early 1930s, an optometrist by the name of A.M. Skeffington theorized that the development of the whole body is important to the development of the visual system, and that the interaction between them is constant and vital. Dr. Arnold Gesell developed Skeffington's theories further in his classic 1949 book, *Vision: Its Development in the Infant and Child*, which illustrated how the child's visual world develops. These ideas form the basis of what we now call vision therapy, or "optometric vision therapy." Vision therapy is an integrated program of techniques and procedures that assist the person in improving all aspects of vision, including general coordination, balance, hand-eye coordination, eye movements, eye teaming (eyes working together), form recognition, visual memory and imagery. I'll be saying more about vision therapy in chapter 9. To find a vision therapy specialist in your area, contact your local Optometric Society by looking under "Optometrists" in the yellow pages of your phone book. You can also contact the College of Optometrists in Vision Development (COVD); their address and phone number are on the list of *Additional Resources* on page 266.

"seeing" and "vision," as we discussed in chapter 3 (see *Seeing Versus Vision*, page 35).

Visual perception develops a little differently in every person, each person's way of seeing being just a little different from the next person's. This is due to all the different stimuli a child receives (or doesn't receive) as he or she grows up. There is an ancient proverb that states: "We see things not as *they* are, but as *we* are." However, there are predictable stages for vision development, and they coincide with the *motor development*—the development of large and small muscle movements—in a child's body.

THE VISUAL-MOTOR CONNECTION

At one time, people believed that the eyes were just two little balls that sat in front of the face to catch light. But, for many years now, we have known that the eyes are an integral part of the central nervous system and are very much influenced by other parts of the body. As the body develops, so do the eyes. Vision is not a separate function; it is integrated with the total "action system" of the child, including posture, manual skills and coordination, intelligence and even personality traits. This is the total vision process.

The development of the muscular system and the visual system together is known as *visual-motor* development. Although vision is one of our "senses," the actions surrounding the visual process are "motor," or muscle-driven. While we are awake, our eyes are constantly responding to shifts of body posture, or they initiate the shifts. Thus, vision influences and is influenced by sensitive patterns of movement of the total person. And, just as it's possible to have poor coordination between two body parts, it is also possible to have poor coordination between the eyes and another body part, or even between one eye and the other.

SEQUENCE OF VISUAL-MOTOR DEVELOPMENT

Patterns of motor development begin in infancy but continue to develop and refine themselves throughout childhood. Any references to ages in this chapter are only averages; it's the sequence of development that counts. If you have any questions about your child's development, consult your pediatrician.

At birth, the infant has only reflexes to work with. However, these reflexes shape the pattern of his motor development.

The first basic motor patterns to develop are the *gross motor* movements. Gross motor refers to the large muscles, such as those in the arms and legs. Gross motor movements are crawling, standing, walking, leg and arm movement, head and neck movements and other large-muscle actions. These movements are necessary for normal growth and development of the baby, enabling him to move in space and use the perceptual tool that is most developed during babyhood—touch.

The baby's exploration and touching experiments eventually lead to the second basic motor pattern: *fine motor* movements. Fine motor movements involve the small muscles and include finger dexterity, toe wiggling, wrist and ankle movements and other subtle motor actions. These are necessary for fine manipulation and, in general, more detailed inspection by the infant of his or her environment. Fine motor coordination is more difficult to achieve if gross motor abilities have not developed on schedule.

Oculomotor skills develop simultaneously with fine and gross motor skills. You may remember from chapter 2 that the eyes are controlled by muscles that surround each eye and are directly connected to the brain (see *How Your Eyes Move*, page 26). Oculomotor development refers to the development of these muscles and their coordination. Efficient eye movement is essential for good eyesight and good vision. The six *extraocular* muscles (muscles outside the eye) have to be able to align each eye with a visual target, and the *intraocular* (inside the eye) muscles must be able to focus the light on the retina in order for the person to see the visual target. In addition, both eyes have to coordinate their movements in order to avoid excess strain or double vision. Once oculomotor development is underway, the child can begin to "feel" with his or her eyes. The process starts slowly. At six to twelve months, touch is still the main avenue of perception. But, once the eye muscles begin to coordinate with each other at about twelve to fifteen months, the majority of sensory input begins to be transferred to the eyes. Eventually the child doesn't have to crawl or walk across the room to identify an object by touch; he can merely look at it and see what it is.

The next phase of development is called *hand-eye coordination*. Hand-eye coordination is the ability of the brain to take in information through the eyes and speedily transfer it to the hands and back again (see *The Eye-Brain Connection*, page 38 to refresh your memory on how visual impulses travel through the brain). This ability takes off around the age of two (although it is present to some degree well before that), but it really continues throughout life. Learning to play a sport at any age is a continuing process of developing hand-eye coordination.

As the visual system develops and oculomotor control increases, the first aspects of *form perception* begin developing. Loosely defined, form perception is the perception of the shapes of objects—and eventually of more abstract things, like words on a page. Form perception, at the earliest stage, starts with the child's perceiving forms by oral investigation. Then, form perception transfers to the fingers, once the fine motor development has been established. Eventually, this transfers to the visual sense, so that the child can recognize forms at a distance based on previous experiences. Advanced form perception includes *figure-ground discrimination*—seeing the main form as different from the background—as well as perception of general shapes, size differentiation, details of configuration and directional orientation. Research has shown that when experienced readers read, they don't perceive individual letters or even words, but rather "forms." Form perception is a complex process for the brain and the visual system to achieve, but it is crucial for good reading.

One aspect of advanced form perception is called *laterality.* Laterality refers to a child's ability to perceive left and right in reference to her own body, and it begins at the age of about five or six. After laterality comes *directionality,* which refers to the child's ability to make left-right distinctions for objects other than herself—say, other people or objects in the room or letters on a piece of paper. This kind of perception usually develops around age six or seven years. If a child can't tell his or her left from right and can't relate that left-right distinction to other objects, then words and letters won't have any meaning. The letter "p" may look the same as a "q" and the "b" the same as a "d," for example. These confusions, called "reversals," are common and expected up to about the age of seven or eight. After that, kids who are still reversing letters need some help in figuring out which way is up!

The next step in the development of visual-motor skills is the area of *visual memory*—the ability to recall visual images, which include everything from a child's list of spelling words to her mother's face to yesterday's dinner. Visual memory begins at about six months but continues to develop as the child matures. It is essential for retention of written material and is, in fact, one measure of a person's intelligence.

LOOK AT THE WHOLE CHILD

Children's eyes are closely influenced by an ever-changing muscle system. Visual defects and deviations from normal may not be apparent if all you're looking for is sharpness of vision that can be measured with an eye chart. Vision problems may make themselves known to you as poor coordination, various forms of awkwardness, poor timing, hesitations and sometimes lack of body movement in a child. If you have any doubts about your child's visual-motor development, don't wait too long to check it out with your pediatrician or eye doctor.

THE EYES BEFORE BIRTH

The first trimester (first three months) of pregnancy is the most critical time for the eyes. The first rudiments of eyes are evident in the fetus at the ripe age of twenty days after conception. Good nutrition, good prenatal care and caution regarding medications and other chemicals (such as alcohol and tobacco) are all important for the development of the fetus's visual system.

There are some things that are genetically determined for the child. Eye color is one of those. All Caucasian babies are born with blue eyes because there is very little pigment accumulated in their irises at birth. As the child grows, more pigment is deposited in the iris, and it begins to look darker. Final eye color depends on how much pigment accumulates. A blue eye simply has less pigment than a brown eye, and a green or hazel eye is somewhere in between.

Another hereditary consideration is color deficiency. The gene for color deficiency is carried on the mother's X chromosome. Females have two X chromosomes, and males have an X and a Y. For a boy to develop color deficiency, he need only have inherited one defective X chromosome from his mother. For a girl to develop color deficiency, she must have *two* defective X chromosomes—one from her mother, and one from her father. This is the reason color deficiency is so much more common in boys than it is in girls.

Nearsightedness (myopia) and crossed eyes do seem to "run in families," but I'm not convinced that genes are entirely to blame for these conditions. A child's genetic makeup may make him or her more or less likely to develop eye problems in any given environment, but it's my belief that the way the child uses his or her eyes in that environment can affect his vision. So, if you're nearsighted, don't throw up your hands and say, "I guess Johnny will be nearsighted too." Start Johnny off right with regular eye exams and good visual habits. Don't wait until it's too late.

NEWBORNS

It is possible to do some eye testing on newborn babies. No, you can't hold an eye chart in front of your infant, but there are certain visual reflexes that are present at birth, and you should know what they are and how to test for them or to have your pediatrician test for them.

Pupil Reflex

The *pupil reflex* to light is present at birth and can easily be tested for by shining a small light into either eye. When you do this, *both* pupils should get smaller. The pupils should be approximately the same size and should stay small as long as the light is still shined into the eye. (Adult eyes react the same way.)

Doll's Eye Reflex

Gently nod your child's head back and forth as you look into his eyes. Notice whether his eyes compensate and try to keep looking at you. They should. This is called the *doll's eye reflex.* (Apparently, the eyes of old-fashioned dolls of the more expensive type swiveled as if to keep looking at you as you turned the doll's head.)

Blink Reflex

The *blink reflex* is the fastest reflex in the body. This is a good indication of how important preserving our eyesight is. Very carefully blow a tiny puff of air at your baby's eyes (gently now!). The eyes should blink immediately.

INFANTS AND TODDLERS

Here are some rough guidelines you can use in evaluating an infant's developing vision. If you have any doubts or questions about your child's eyes, your pediatrician or eye doctor is the one to see.

The one-month-old: At one month, the baby will probably stare blankly around the room, although a bright light or window light should attract her attention. Occasionally there will be a little following of an object brought in front of her face. Contrary to popular belief, babies are not "born blind." However, the macula of the retina is not completely developed at birth, so the infant's visual acuity is poor. (It gradually improves until we expect 20/20 visual acuity at about the age of five or six years.)

The two-month-old: At two months, you should notice a few more eye movements in your infant, although they will still be limited. The child will start to realize what the parents' faces look like and may be able to distinguish them from just any face. This is the first indication of visual memory. Some authorities believe that babies are "programmed" to recognize faces better than any other kind of visual pattern. In terms of evolution and infant survival, this makes good sense.

The three-month-old: At three months, the child should be able to follow a dangling object from one end of his visual gaze to the other, although the eye movements may be unsteady. If he gets hold of a rattle, you may notice him looking at it occasionally. At this stage, the baby prefers using his mouth to his eyes for investigational purposes. But, since any kind of investigation the baby does is important for his developing vision, be sure to keep plenty of clean, harmless toys close by. Gross motor development at this point usually appears as lifting of the head and chest when lying prone, as well as kicking of the legs in random movements.

The four-month-old: The four-month-old child will stop occasionally to visually inspect things, such as her hand or a toy. Her head movements should be more pronounced and should be more independent of eye movements. This is the early stage of oculomotor development.

The five-month-old: The five-month-old child may try to keep an object in sight as it is brought to his mouth; he releases this fixation in an unsteady manner.

The six-month-old: At six months, the child should be able to follow an object for a few seconds, although she may lose it to follow another one. More fluid eye movements are evident now. Interest in objects across the room should be encouraged to help the baby learn about size and distance. Give the child plenty of room to crawl and explore. Gross motor development should be much more apparent as movement expands. The baby rolls around and attempts to lift herself upright. Fine motor development is coming along too; the baby may attempt to manipulate a toy, and her hands are becoming more independent. Movements are beginning to integrate all parts of the body, matching sight with other kinds of perception (such as touch and hearing).

The seven-month-old: At seven months the infant will noticeably improve eye movements, specifically convergence.

He can now converge his eyes to inspect a toy at close range, although he may lose this fixation momentarily and then regain it. Hand-eye coordination begins its refinement as the child feels more comfortable with fine motor coordination, such a lifting a cup to inspect it. Large muscles will allow him to sit up and start creeping.

The eight-month-old: At eight months the child begins to manipulate objects with more sophistication, turning objects about in his hands to explore them visually. He may hold one toy while manipulating another. He becomes more aware of the space outside his reach and will watch others across the room. He should be well into crawling now. During the second six months of life, infants need plenty of crawling opportunities. Crawling is an important stage of development that allows the child to fully integrate all of his major muscle groups with his perceptual abilities—at ground level. Unfortunately, many parents are too anxious to have little Johnny walking and want to hurry him through the crawling stage. Don't rush the child. I've seen many learning-disabled children with behavior problems walked at an early age without the benefit of crawling.

The ten-month-old: At ten months there is an increase in the ease of movement of the child's head and trunk. Vertical surfaces become intriguing as the child prepares to stand. Eye muscles and large muscles work together in this process. The child now starts to see the "whole" of objects, which is rudimentary form perception.

The one-year-old: The one-year-old should be mastering her vertical orientation. Walking with assistance and standing alone temporarily indicate that gross motor development is proceeding on schedule. Visually, the child refines eye movements; she may have unusual facial expressions at times as part of this process. Smooth, easy visual pursuit of objects and increased mobility of the eyes become apparent. Eye movements are now not necessarily associated with head movements.

The first three years: During the first three years, the child begins to refine his or her eye movements, hand-eye coordination, visual perception, his ability to see contrasts and forms and his ability to focus his eyes for near and distance vision. The more visual input he receives, the more opportunity the child has to use his or her eyes and brain to see. It is at this time that the basic visual perception patterns are formed. Some optometrists are able to do perception development testing, so don't hesitate to get the examination if you have any doubts about your child's vision. Don't forget: *Your child can't make that decision; only you can.*

Cover Test

As soon as your child is able to focus on an object for several seconds at a time (usually at about age three), you can try this test to see whether she can use her eyes together properly.

1. Have your child look at one particular object that will hold his or her attention (try entrancing her with a small flashlight inserted into a finger puppet).

2. Cover one of her eyes while you look at the other eye. Make sure she stays focused on the object, not on your hand.

3. Did the uncovered eye move when the cover was put in place? Try this a few times to be sure. If your child had both eyes focused on the object to begin with, she shouldn't need to refocus when one eye is covered. In other words, there shouldn't be any movement of the uncovered eye.

4. Uncover both eyes again and let the child focus on the object.

5. Cover the other eye (the one you previously left uncovered), and watch the uncovered one; any movement to relocate the object? If she was using both eyes to focus, there shouldn't be any readjustment necessary.

You are testing the child's ability to use both eyes together properly. If you saw any movement of the uncovered eye when the cover was placed over the other one, consult an optometrist to verify the finding. At this early age any binocular (two-eyed) dysfunction should be easy to rectify.

THE PRESCHOOL YEARS

Between the ages of two and five, the normal child's eyes, in conjunction with the rest of his body and brain, make great strides toward adult visual capabilities and are getting ready for the challenge of reading and writing.

The two-year-old: By the age of two the child should have good footing—good enough to be able to run without falling (well, at least some of the time). He should be using his eyes more responsively, watching what he does as he does it. Eyes and hands are less closely associated now than they were earlier; he'll usually look, then act instead of doing both simultaneously. Whirling disks and brightly colored objects are quite a source of fascination at this age. Small objects might be studied with more intensity than before, a sure sign of increased visual discrimination. Attention span at this age is about seven minutes.

The three-year-old: The three-year-old is definitely more organized in his actions than the two-year-old. Hand-eye activities are more unified: He will color within the lines of a picture, and he can use his hands more freely without riveting his eyes to them. His eyes may take a more directive role, often not accompanied by head movements anymore, leading where they had previously been following. An increase in space orientation should become evident; the child knows where he is and knows more about where other objects are in relation to him. Attention span increases to about nine minutes now.

The four-year-old: In general, by the time the child reaches four, you should be noticing a definite expansion of motor development. The child has bursts of racing, hopping, jumping, skipping and climbing. The child seems to be saying, "Look out world, here I come!" Motor patterns show a tendency for symmetry, using both hands and recognizing two halves as a whole picture. Eye teaming becomes more obvious. There is now a loose organization of the visual system that allows the child's eyes to work together and to accommodate better. Attention span now is about twelve to fifteen minutes.

The five-year-old: The five-year-old's coordination has reached a new maturity with a greater ease and control of general body

A Child's-Eye View

Let's say that right now you're sitting on a chair at a desk, reading. You are well aware of the distance from you to the desk, the desk to the wall, the room to the rest of the house. If you shift your attention from this book to your refrigerator, you remain aware of the book's location so you can return to it after eating without spending ten minutes looking for it.

Now think of how a preschool child relates to these things. Each time he shifts attention from one object to another, he forgets where the other objects are. It's more than just poor memory; it's actually an inability to relate spatial locations in his visual world until the age of about five or six. If, for some reason, a child is a little late in catching on to these spatial relationships and can't keep them straight in his head, he can't make any progress because new experiences keep crowding in; new expectations are made as a new age is reached and he has not yet conquered the old ones.

Now, what does all this have to do with a child's vision and his achievement? Just this: If a perceptual "lag" persists into his school years, he may have trouble with arithmetic and spelling. He won't understand that $2 + 2 = 4$ because that is a relationship among four different objects. He may have trouble remembering that the two letters "g" and "o" spell "go" because that is true only if they are arranged in that particular order. A child who can't tell left from right (a spatial relationship) might come out with "og." This may be the basis for the reversals commonly seen in poor achievers and children with learning disabilities. As an adult, these problems may be difficult to understand unless you experienced them yourself.

It's important to be aware of perception from a child's point of view. If you do, it will be easier to find ways for him to catch on to what should be accomplished. This can easily be achieved by giving him or her a tremendous amount of experiences with shapes, movement and distances and regular eye examinations starting at the age of three (earlier if you suspect problems). Then all they need is love.

activity. Movements are more refined, and so is hand-eye coordination. The child moves with more deliberation and a finer coordination of movements. Her eyes can fix on something more easily now, and the mechanics of focusing are now developed to the point where focusing is more accurate. Attention span increases to thirty minutes.

THE SCHOOL YEARS

School and vision—the two words are practically synonymous. School is for learning, and at least 80 percent of learning is mediated through vision. Everything your child has developed before now will come into play during school. And there will not be a more demanding test of visual abilities than at school.

Unfortunately, four out of ten grade school children in the United States are visually handicapped for adequate school achievement. Visual handicaps include not only seeing a blur while looking at the blackboard, but can be poor oculomotor coordination, crossed or "lazy" eyes, focusing insufficiency, perceptual problems or developmental lags.

Let's take a look at a few of the things that a child has to use his eyes for in school.

Near vision: This is the ability to see clearly at a fourteen- to sixteen-inch reading distance with both eyes.

Distance vision: This is the ability to see at least a twenty-foot distance with sharpness and very little effort.

Accommodation: This is the ability to accommodate for near tasks easily (with no effort). This process must be done with comfort and must be maintained for long periods of time.

Focusing flexibility: This is the ability to alternate between distance and near vision quickly and effortlessly.

Binocular coordination: This is the ability to make both eyes work together as a team while looking at distance or near. Tiring, double vision, poor reading and headaches are a few signs of poor binocular coordination.

Adequate field of vision: This is the ability to see up, down, left and right while focusing at one spot. This saves unnecessary head and eye movements and is crucial for reading.

These are only some of the visual abilities that are needed for good performance in school. Please keep in mind that *a school vision screening is not an eye examination.* Most schools just do the standard eye-chart test that is usually required by state law. By now, you should be aware that there are many other problems that can arise. Often, by the time the child's distance vision starts to decline enough to show up on the Snellen test, the problem is well on its way to becoming a permanent handicap. Distance vision is usually the last thing to go wrong, so a complete vision exam with an eye doctor is necessary to find any other problems first. Make a complete vision exam part of your back-to-school routine. And, if at any time, your child is having vision problems or is in the lower third of his or her class, a complete vision exam is in order.

Know Your ABC's

Here are the ABC's of signs and symptoms that may signal vision trouble during the school years. Look for them in your child.

A — APPEARANCE OF EYES
Crossed or pointing out, up or down
Red
Watery
Encrusted lids
Frequent styes

B — BEHAVIOR
Squinting or closing of one eye
Rigid body posture
Avoids close work
Rocks back and forth
Head turning
Excessive head movement
Too close to work
Uses finger to read
Blinks much and with effort
Rubs eyes during or after short periods of reading

C – COMPLAINTS
    Blurred vision
    Headaches
    Nausea or dizziness
    Burning or itching eyes
    Seeing double
    Tires quickly while reading

High-Risk Ages

Vision problems can develop at any age, but there do seem to be certain times during a child's school years when they are more likely to occur.

Second grade: Sudden increases in myopia seem to occur in the second grade, the time when the child is learning to read and the demand for close work is greatly increased over any previous year.

Fourth grade: Now, instead of learning to read, the child is reading to learn. This means that a possibly unmastered skill must now be used to investigate new areas of learning. It's as if you had just begun learning French and suddenly had to study nuclear physics in the new language. The result of this kind of stress and more intense close work is often myopia.

Seventh grade: Junior high school is a time for a physical growth spurt combined with a tremendously increased demand for near work: a recipe for myopia.

Ninth grade: Around the ninth grade, reading assignments pile on and pressures to achieve in school increase. Teenagers may adapt to the stress by developing myopia (if they haven't done so already). If vision problems go uncorrected, a teenager may give up on schoolwork and show declining achievement.

All of these periods of high stress require a good vision exam—which should be done every year anyway. So, when September rolls around and you're buying the new clothes and supplies for school and getting a medical exam and dental checkup, don't forget about the one school supply that needs to be in the best working order: *vision.*

Special Problems

Here are some specific problems that occur in children and can be much improved or entirely corrected by prompt intervention.

MYOPIA (NEARSIGHTEDNESS) IN CHILDREN

Myopia, or nearsightedness, is the most common refractive error in humans, affecting over 32 percent of the population in the United States. It usually starts in childhood if it's going to start at all, worsens until early adulthood and then usually stabilizes.

How It Happens

As you may remember from chapter 2 (see *Nearsighted or Farsighted?*, page 22), myopia means an image is being focused in front of the retina. This misplacement of focus can be caused by the eye being too long so that the retina is farther back than it should be, by the eye's lens staying focused for near or by a corneal curvature that causes the light to focus too soon. It can be corrected with glasses or contact lenses that force the image farther back so that it lands on the retina.

It's been believed for a long time now that myopia is inherited, and I don't deny that heredity may be a factor in this condition. But, it's probably not the whole story, because myopia is much more prevalent in people and societies where a lot of close work is done. Studies have found, for example, that myopia is almost nonexistent in uneducated societies (such as early Eskimos or some African tribes) and that myopia increases in proportion to the amount of education in any given society. In other words, the more reading and near-point work the society does, the higher the incidence of myopia.

In a similar vein, studies have been conducted with Navy submariners, who are submerged for months at a time in a space where their maximum viewing distance is about eight feet. The studies showed an increase in myopia during these extended periods of confinement.

Dr. Francis Young of Washington University has done similar research with monkeys. Dr. Young kept rhesus monkeys in confined areas during various developmental periods of their early life. The shorter the maximum viewing distance and the longer the confinement, the more myopia the monkeys developed.

So what does this say about the way our eyes develop? As with any biological system, our visual system will change in response to stress. While reading, your eyes are focused at a close distance—usually about fourteen to sixteen inches. The eye accomplishes this focusing through the process of accommodation (see *How You Focus Your Eyes*, page 18). If this posture is maintained for long periods of time without a rest, the eyes slowly adapt to the position in order to reduce the stress on the muscles controlling each eye's lens. Once adapted, the eyes can see more clearly up close with less effort. It's as if the muscles get comfortably "stuck" in the near-focus position. To make matters worse, when the eye muscles work constantly to accommodate for near work, they cause some increased pressure to build up in the eye. Eventually, this pressure causes the eyeball itself to lengthen (which relieves the pressure), moving the retina farther back from the lens than it originally was. The result of all this? Myopia. When the myopic eye relaxes the accommodation and attempts to refocus for distance, the image is blurred because it is too far forward of the retina. This process doesn't happen by just reading steadily for a night or two. It's a gradual adaptation that your eyes go through as they react to the strain of overwork.

As you might expect, myopia increases in children as they spend more and more of their time focused for near-vision activities. About 1.6 percent of children entering school in the United States have some degree of myopia. That figure grows to 4.4 percent for seven- and eight-year-olds, 8.7 percent for nine- and ten-year-olds, 12.5 percent for eleven- and twelve-year-olds and 14.3 percent for thirteen- and fourteen-year-olds. We used to say that the progression (worsening) of myopia stabilized at about twenty-one or twenty-two years of age. However, over the past ten years, eye-care professionals have seen more and more myopia progressing well into the late twenties or even thirties. The reason? We're not quite sure, but computers are almost certainly one of the culprits. They require constant near-point focus, and more and more adults are spending more and more time in front of them (see *Near Vision at Work*, page 176).

What to Do About It

There's probably no escape from activities that require near-point focus. Consider all that we do with our eyes at the near point: reading, writing, drawing, typing, painting, sewing, crocheting, tying shoe laces and even cooking and eating, to name just a few. And then there are those intermediate-distance tasks, such as playing the piano (or most musical instruments), shopping, card playing, watching television and a variety of hobbies. During the grade school years a child will read the equivalent of about seven hundred books. It's not hard to see why so many people develop myopia. Have you ever seen a lawyer, for example, who doesn't wear glasses? (If you have, he's probably wearing contacts!)

So, what can be done about all this? Well, you could stay away from all those near-point activities, but that's not too practical. So, first, make sure your child has a complete vision exam from an optometrist or ophthalmologist who performs near-vision tests. Many doctors omit these because they take longer to do and evaluate than simple tests of distance vision. Also, at home, be sure there's enough indirect light for homework, and do not have a desk for a child that faces a wall. You want her to be able to look up and focus for distance from time to time. Have your child do about twenty to thirty minutes of reading, then take two minutes or so to look far away or close her eyes. Reading distance should be kept at fourteen to sixteen inches—no closer! (*See* illustration, page 63.) If the child complains about not being able to read at this distance, then something is wrong and a full exam is indicated. In short, give the eyes a chance to relax when doing a lot of close work, and have routine eye exams to be sure everything is working properly.

If glasses are prescribed for your child's myopia, they won't "cure" him, but they certainly will make distance vision easier. He should, however, take off his glasses for reading and other near-point activities, since wearing them for those activities only forces his eyes to accommodate more and may hasten the progression of the myopia. Sometimes we even prescribe bifocals for children with one clear section (for near vision) and one prescription section (for distance vision) in each eyeglass lens. That way, kids don't have to take their glasses on and off for distance and near activities.

If he's old enough, your child should participate in choosing his glasses—with help from you and the optician, of course. Choose a sturdy frame that fits properly even though you may be tempted to get one that allows for growth. Plastic lenses are less likely to break than glass ones; on the other hand, they

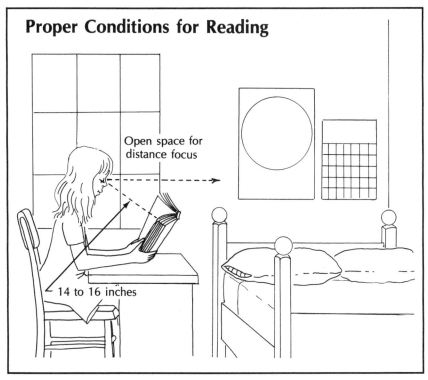

Proper Conditions for Reading

Open space for distance focus

14 to 16 inches

When a child reads, the book should be kept at fourteen to sixteen inches from the eyes. Equally important, the child should be able to look up from reading every twenty to thirty minutes and focus into the distance. For this reason, it's best not to have a desk or reading area that faces a wall. (All this applies to adults also!)

scratch more easily and will probably have to be replaced sooner. (For more information about choosing glasses, see *Choosing Frames for Children*, page 125.)

STRABISMUS ('CROSSED' EYES)

Remember when you were a child in grade school? There was probably one boy or girl who appeared strange because when she or he looked at you, he wasn't really looking at you! You probably couldn't figure out which eye to look at. For the 2 percent of this nation's children who have crossed eyes, growing up can be socially, as well as visually, painful.

Strabismus

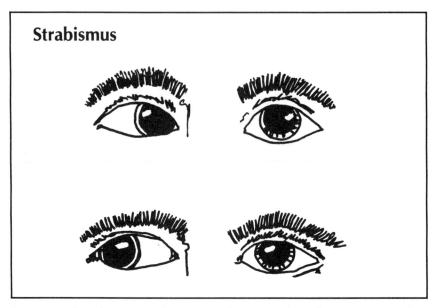

A person with strabismus may have an eye that is turned up, down, in or out. When an eye is turned toward the nasal side, it's usually called "crossed." When an eye is turned toward the temporal side, it's usually called "wall-eyed." Children usually have the kind of strabismus in which an eye turns toward the nasal side.

Strabismus (stra-BIZ-muss) is the technical term for crossed eyes. Actually, "crossed" is somewhat of a misnomer, because an eye can be turned up, down, in or out—they're all called "strabismus" (*see* illustration above). When an eye is turned toward the nose—toward the *nasal* side—it's usually called "crossed." When an eye is turned toward the ear—called the *temporal* side—it's called "wall-eyed." In children, strabismus usually involves an eye that is turned nasally. About half of those people who have strabismus were born with it. Somewhere along the line, the eye-brain hookup got "wired" wrong. Some authorities believe that there is a hereditary predisposition for strabismus; I've seen it occur occasionally in the same family.

What causes strabismus? Believe it or not, we don't really know for sure in many cases. Some cases of strabismus are induced by a poor visual environment—for example, by isolating an infant in a dark room or by keeping an infant positioned with the same eye closer to the mattress. Your eyes are made to receive light; that's how they function best. The more they are used, the better they develop. The more visual stimulation presented to a child, the more visual experience he can have, which should lead to better visual development. If this stimulation is deficient or is limited to one side, then the visual system will not develop symmetrically.

It is important to remember that your eyes are directly connected to the brain and that they are controlled from there. And so are the six sets of eye muscles attached to the eyeball. They control where you aim your eyes.

Years ago, doctors thought that the turning of an eye was a purely mechanical error caused by an eye muscle that was too long or too short. All they had to do was surgically shorten or move a muscle in order to straighten out the eye. Sound logical? Well, maybe. But consider this: An eye muscle is a hundred times as strong as it needs to be to turn an eyeball. Why, then, can't it just pull the eye in the right direction without benefit of surgery?

The answer turns out to be that strabismus is usually a problem of eye-brain coordination, not just of muscles that are too short or too long. We can test the eye muscles of a child with strabismus and find that they are in perfect working order—but the child still can't aim her eyes in the same direction.

Some physicians still routinely recommend eye surgery to correct strabismus. I usually advise against surgery for strabismus, although it does help in some extreme cases. Most of the time, I find, such surgery doesn't really correct the problem; it only makes the eyes *appear* to be aimed at the same point. If you have received a recommendation to have this type of surgery done, I would recommend a second opinion with an ophthalmologist who specializes in this procedure and also one with an optometrist who uses nonsurgical theraputic techniques to teach the eyes to work together.

Nonsurgical Treatment for Strabismus

There are several ways to treat strabismus without surgery.

Occluding vision in the good eye: One way of treating strabismus is to force the child to use the turned eye by covering the "good" eye for prescribed periods of time. The good eye can be covered with a patch or with an opaque lens in a pair of eyeglasses. Vision in the good eye can also be occluded with the use of eye drops that blur the vision in that eye. You have to be careful not to obscure vision from the good eye for too many

Is She Really Cross-Eyed?

You may look at your very young child one day and think she looks cross-eyed. It is common for young children to have a cross-eyed appearance even when there is nothing wrong with their eye alignment because of skin folds around the eyes that hide part of the whites of the eyes, and an undeveloped nasal bone, which gives that area a flattened shape. This is called *pseudostrabismus* (*see* illustration, page 67). To see whether the eyes are really turned in, lift the skin of the nose away from the eyes and look straight at the child. Do the eyes still look crossed? If so, try this test. Have your child look at a penlight as you bring it close to her eyes. As you get close to her eyes with the penlight (about a foot away), you should see the reflection of the penlight on each iris of her eyes. The reflection should be slightly to the nasal side on each iris and in the same place on each iris. This is because her eyes are moving toward each other to focus on the light. If your child has an eye that is turned nasally, the reflection of the light will be more temporal on that eye than on the normal eye; it will not be at the same point in relation to the iris on both eyes. If a child has an eye that is turned temporally, the reflection of the light will be more nasal in the turned eye. If you have any doubts about whether or not your child has strabismus, consult your eye doctor or pediatrician. If strabismus is suspected, the back of the eye must be examined by a doctor because, in rare cases, strabismus can be caused by a tumor of the eye.

hours of the day, or you may risk losing vision in the good eye. You'll need to see a pediatric ophthalmologist for guidance with this kind of treatment.

Using glasses: Sometimes childhood strabismus is caused by farsightedness (hyperopia). The child tries to compensate for his or her farsightedness by overconverging the eyes, so that they both turn in too much. This kind of strabismus should be treated with glasses that correct the hyperopia.

Exercises and activities: Here are some things you can do to prevent or treat strabismus in an infant or child.

Pseudostrabismus

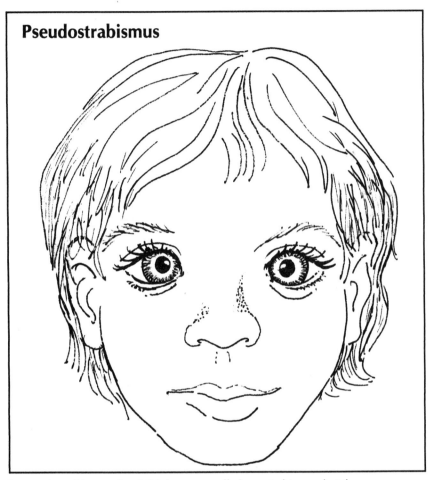

In pseudostrabismus, the child does not really have strabismus, but the eyes may appear crossed because of skin folds around them that hide some of the white of the eye. A broad, flat nasal bridge may contribute to the illusion. You may be able to tell if there is any real strabismus just by lifting the skin away from the nasal side of the eyes and seeing if the eyes still look crossed. As a further test, you can try shining a penlight into the child's eyes and seeing if the reflection of the light is at the same point on each iris. It should be if the eyes are properly aligned (*see* box on page 66 for complete instructions).

• Have your infant lie on her back and stand directly in front of her. Grasp both the child's wrists and slowly pull her up. Repeat this procedure a few times as if it were a game so as not to tire the child. This exercise will help the child's neck muscles to develop properly. Good control of the neck muscles aids in the development of binocular vision.

• Hold your infant in the air and attract his attention to your face. Then, gradually bring the child closer to you, which will cause his eyes to converge. Bring the child all the way to your nose and make a funny sound when your noses touch; then lift the child away again. Try this a few times as if it were a game. This game will develop the child's ability to converge the eyes effectively.

• Use a boldly striped black and white material as a drape over the edge when leaving an infant to play in her crib. This will stimulate the child's visual development.

• Line up four or five toys that squeak. Sit across from your child and squeeze the farthest one to one side. As soon as the child looks at it and atetmpts to grasp it, squeeze the farthest one on the other side of the row. Encourage the child to look at this one. Then, as he goes for it, squeeze the first one again. Repeat this only as long as the child feels it's a game and doesn't become frustrated or irrritable. This game will stimulate the eyes to move in both directions.

• Have the child look through a stereoscopic viewer, such as the one made by View-Master®, at three-dimensional slides. These are available with cartoon characters, animals and other fun things to look at. Ask the child whether the character or animal looks as if its "sticking out" at her. The child will get this three-dimensional effect only if she is using binocular vision.

• Have older children try the exercises I recommend for binocular coordination in chapter 9 (see *Brock String Exercise*, *Convergence Stimulation* and *Convergence Relaxation*, pages 158, 160 and 162).

Surgical Treatment for Strabismus

Surgical treatment for strabismus is beneficial in some cases. Pediatric ophthalmologists sometimes choose to operate on the muscles of *both* eyes, even though only one eye may be turned. This is because they've found that when only one eye is operated on, it may cause the other eye to "follow" it. For example, if a nasally turned eye is operated on and pulled temporally, it may cause the other eye to become turned nasally. The operation that is often performed to straighten a nasally turned eye weakens the power of the muscle on the nasal side of both eyes. This is done by moving the muscles further back on each eye, thus loosening the tension on the muscles.

Another procedure for strabismus involves only the turned eye. If the eye is turned nasally, the muscle on the nasal side is moved back, as in the other operation, to reduce the tension on that side. Then, the muscle on the temporal side is shortened, which increases the tension on that side and turns the eye toward the temporal side. To turn an eye toward the nasal side, the opposite procedure can be done; the muscle on the temporal side can be moved back, while the muscle on the nasal side can be shortened.

AMBLYOPIA

If the visual information to one eye is distorted or dissimilar from the other eye in any way, the brain will receive two images that are very different from each other. The child may experience double vision under these circumstances. Since this is obviously an undesirable condition, the brain will "turn off" one of those images in order to see one image again. That one image will then be coming from only one eye. This turning off of the input from one eye can occur when strabismus causes the eyes to point at two different objects rather than the same one. (One of the main reasons to treat strabismus is to prevent amblyopia.) It can also occur if the two eyes are dissimilar in the way they handle refraction—for example, if one eye is myopic and the other astigmatic. If the situation exists for a long time, the eye that is not being used will adapt to seeing that way: poorly. After some time, the best obtainable vision will not be as good as was once possible, even if the proper correcting lens is placed before the eye. This condition of having a perfectly healthy eye that cannot be fully corrected to 20/20 is called *amblyopia* (am-blee-OH-pee-ah). The eye's vision has been "sacrificed" to preserve the child's ability to function.

Amblyopia affects about four million people in the United States, and there is no definitive medical treatment for it. The only treatment is to try to encourage the eye to see clearly. Amblyopia can be prevented almost 100 percent of the time if it is detected early enough (during early childhood) and if the cause is effectively treated. The strabismus or other eye condition that is causing one eye to "turn off" must be treated so that both eyes start working together.

One additional note: If your child has one good eye and one that is amblyopic, I strongly suggest that he or she wear protective eyewear at all times. You never know when some object may come too close for comfort. A pair of "plano" or nonprescription, unbreakable, polycarbonate lenses are the best protection you could have. Ask your optician about these lenses (see *Flying Objects*, page 198 for more information).

DYSLEXIA

Oftentimes we come across a child who doesn't seem to be reading even though he's intelligent and motivated. The child "wants" to learn and seems to try as hard as possible. Teachers say that he is an intelligent boy who "doesn't apply himself," whatever that means!

The term *dyslexia* was developed some years ago to describe a set of symptoms relating to the inability of some people to read and understand written language despite normal intelligence and educational opportunities.

Early research in dyslexia looked for a single factor to explain the disorder. Some experts thought the problem had to do with visual acuity or binocular coordination, while others related the disorder to everything from an inner-ear condition to psychological difficulties, faulty educational methods and brain damage. As with most complex problems, it is now apparent that there are no simple answers to the puzzle of dyslexia. There are probably different causes for the symptoms in different children, although there is now some pretty hard evidence that certain areas of the brain develop more slowly in dyslexic children than they do in other children.

Research in dyslexia continues to investigate the role of the visual system. The visual system is almost certainly involved in some way with the problem, although exactly *how* it is involved is not clear. Dyslexic children usually have good visual acuity, although they seem to have difficulty focusing their eyes. Interestingly, children with *severe* strabismus usually do not have difficulty reading, because they have managed to suppress the image from the severely affected eye and are reading with the good eye. Children with *mild* strabismus, on the other hand, may be dyslexic, because they're struggling to fuse two different images from their two different eyes. In the 1980s, psychologist Helen Irlen found another visual problem related to dyxlexia; her findings suggested that at least some dyslexics were extremely sensitive to light. She developed a treatment for dyslexia

Irlen Lenses

In the 1980s, Dr. Helen Irlen, a psychologist, developed a theory that at least some dyslexic people had an unusual sensitivity to light that was interfering with their reading ability. According to Irlen's theory, they were using their night vision all the time, which created some visual distortion when they tried to read black letters on a white background. Irlen called this problem the *scotopic sensitivity syndrome.*

She began experimenting with light-filtering, colored lenses for dyslexics to use while reading. These are now called "Irlen lenses." The approach used by the Irlen Institute is, first, to have a complete vision examination to rule out any refractive problems—that is, making sure the child can see clearly. Next comes an evaluation to determine the exact visual distortions being experienced relating to light sensitivity, visual resolution (blur), span of focus and sustained focus during the reading process. Lastly, the distortions are minimized or eliminated by selecting the appropriate tint from a range of 150 color possiblities.

For more information about the Irlen lenses, write to or call the Irlen Institute. The address and phone number can be found in the list of *Additional Resources* on page 266.

that makes use of special light-filtering lenses, now called *Irlen lenses* (*see* box above).

If you suspect that your child may have dyslexia, it's best to get a thorough vision exam as well as educational testing that includes an assessment of the child's visual-motor development.

What to Look for When Children Read

In evaluating your child for dyslexia and for vision problems that may affect reading, here are some signs to look for when watching and listening to children read. Remember that many of these problems are normal at certain stages and that every child develops at his or her own pace. Some things to look for are:

- poor reading comprehension
- loses place often during reading

- short attention span in reading
- too frequently omits words
- writes uphill or downhill on paper
- rereads or skips lines unknowingly
- fails to recognize same word in next sentence
- mistakes words with same or similar beginnings
- fails to visualize what is read
- repeatedly confuses left-right directions
- orients drawings poorly on page
- loses interest too quickly

Be sure to get a thorough vision exam to make sure your child gets off to a good start in reading.

YOUR CHILD'S EYE EXAM

If you've taken your child to a good eye doctor, he or she will be able to explain any visual difficulty of your child's so that you can understand the problem. Don't hesitate to ask any questions that might come up. This chapter may have helped you decide which questions to ask. In any case, be sure you understand the following aspects of the exam:

Visual acuity: First, you should know your child's visual acuity. Although the 20/20 is only an arbitrary figure, it still gives an idea of how close to "normal" a child's vision is.

Refractive errors: You should understand your child's myopia, hyperopia or astigmatism, if any of these are present, and how these conditions will be corrected.

Health of the eyes: Next, you should be informed of the external and internal health of the eyes. This is a very basic and necessary finding; eyes must be healthy to see well.

Eye-brain coordination: The doctor should tell you about any special eye-brain coordination problems, such as strabismus or amblyopia. A treatment plan should be devised.

Focusing ability and flexibility: The doctor should see whether the child can maintain his or her focus for near or distance vision and switch back and forth easily from near to far and back again.

Binocular efficiency: This is a critical area in the child's vision. Can the child maintain binocular fixation on a certain point for a sustained period of time? How is his depth perception?

Color vision: The child's color vision should be tested and explained.

Perceptual and developmental tests: If a child is having some difficulty in school, a series of perceptual or developmental tests may be recommended. Make sure you understand the purpose and results of these tests. If vision therapy is prescribed, it too should be thoroughly explained.

Glasses and contact lenses: Be sure you and the child know exactly when to wear the prescribed glasses (for which activities) and how to care for them, and how to care for, insert and remove contact lenses.

GROWING UP WITH TV

It's no surprise to anyone that some children want to spend as much time watching TV as they spend at school. Television has been a powerful influence on kids (and adults) for several generations. Since watching TV involves eye use, many people have been concerned with the visual effects of extended viewing. A few studies have been done in this area, and some interesting conclusions have been reached. Here are answers to some of the more frequently asked questions about television and vision.

Q. How does watching TV affect the eyes?
A. There's less focus strain involved in viewing television than in doing close work like reading or computer work. However, close concentration and staring at the television screen over an excessive period of time may result in general fatigue and tired eyes.

Q. Can a room be too bright for comfortable viewing?
A. Yes. Excessively bright room lighting tends to reduce con-

trast on the screen and "wash out" the picture. No lights should be placed where glare or reflections will be seen in or near the television screen.

Q. How can one best adjust the lighting?

A. It is better to adjust the brightness and contrast of the television picture after the proper room lights have been turned on. Adapt the set to room lighting, not vice versa.

Q. Should you watch TV in a totally darkened room?

A. No!! The contrast between the screen and the surrounding area is too great for comfortable and efficient vision. When the room is softly illuminated, this undesirable high contrast is kept to a minimum.

Q. How close should you be to the screen?

A. Picture details will appear much sharper and better defined if the screen is viewed from a distance that is at least five times the diagonal dimension of the screen (*see* illustration, page 75). For example, if you have a nineteen-inch screen—measured from the lower left to the upper right corner or the lower right to the upper left corner—it should be viewed from a distance of at least eight feet. Nearsighted kids are the ones most likely to persist in sitting two or three feet from the screen. (There's really no such thing as sitting too far from the screen.)

Q. Does radiation come out of a TV screen?

A. There is some radiation emitted from both black-and-white and color TV screens, and more is emitted from a color screen. At this time, it does not seem to pose a health hazard, although many experts think you should not sit too close to a color screen. Stick with the distance recommended—five times the diagonal dimension of the screen—for safety as well as comfort.

Q. Does body posture affect viewing comfort?

A. Yes. Watching television in a twisted or leaning position will cause one eye to see much more than the other eye. This will lead to eyestrain because the vision is not balanced equally between the eyes. An erect, straight-ahead position is best suited for television watching.

With a little common sense and these few facts, you and your child can learn to live with TV and make the most of the experience. Junk-food commercials aside, television has much to offer for the growth and development of children.

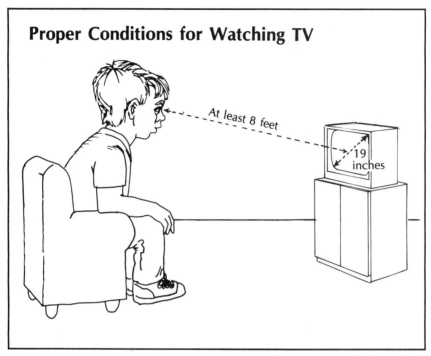

Proper Conditions for Watching TV

At least 8 feet

19 inches

The child should sit at a distance from the TV screen that is at least five times the diagonal dimension of the screen (for example, ninety-five inches, or about eight feet, away from a nineteen-inch screen). He should not watch TV in a twisted or leaning position, which will cause one eye to see more than the other and result in eyestrain. Room lighting should neither be excessively bright nor completely dark. Soft room lighting is best.

GOOD VISION— HOW PARENTS CAN HELP

If you've read this chapter, you know that a child's vision is an integral part of her whole development and goes hand-in-hand with the maturation of her large and small muscles and her brain. Most of the time, vision develops properly and on schedule. Once in a while, it seems delayed or deficient, which usually means you'll need to seek help from your pediatrician, eye doctor or school-associated professionals. Even when vision does seem to be developing properly, there are things you as a parent can do to ensure that it stays on track. Try some of the activities on the next few pages for good fun and good vision.

Developing coordination: Coordination is the ability to move one's body in a controlled manner.

• Let your child crawl over, under and around chairs or tables, watching for sharp corners.

• Play "Mother, May I?" with your child. Use running, hopping, crawling and jumping skills in the game.

• Ask your child to walk backwards or sideways when you're on walks together.

• Have your child hop on his or her left foot, then on the right. Have the child hop on both feet or run in place to music while you count to ten.

• Have your child jump forward or backward over a line or crack.

• Have your child run on tiptoes and then stand on tiptoes for ten seconds.

• Play "Simon Says" with your child. Use directions that include the terms "right" and "left." Encourage any activity that requires and reinforces the right-left terminology.

• Practice naming parts of the body while touching them.

• Bounce a ball to your child. Have your child catch and bounce the ball back.

• Teach skipping by having the child hop forward on the right foot and then bring the left foot up to the right.

• Use a two-inch by four-inch balance beam. Have the child walk along it with arms out or clasped behind the body. Also try different techniques and games on the beam, including walking back and forth with eyes closed.

Developing visual-motor control: Visual-motor control is the ability to control the movements of the small-muscle groups in conjunction with the eye muscles.

• Have your child make scrap pictures from material — string, buttons, beads, shells or anything lying around.

• Draw a line pattern on a piece of paper while your child follows the pattern with his or her finger.

• Practice turning pages.

• Have your child string pieces of macaroni as if they were beads.

• Fold a piece of paper into many parts. Open it up and have your child draw along the folded lines.

• Help your child practice tying knots and bows in shoes or pieces of string.

• Put some cornmeal or sand in a tray and have your child practice drawing shapes or letters in it.

• Write letters with dots and have your child trace over them.

• Have your child color in the "o's" in a newspaper article.

Developing visual perception: Visual perception is the ability to perceive such things as colors, shapes, sizes, letter forms and words.

• Place some objects on the floor. Have your child arrange them according to size or color.

• Play "smaller-larger." As an example, ask the child to "find something smaller than your head but larger than your hand."

• Talk about colors.

• Have your child help separate teaspoons and tablespoons.

• Have your child measure the size of different things— furniture, paper, rooms and so on.

• Give your child a piece of string and have him or her find five things longer and five things shorter than it is.

• Draw arrows in different directions on a card. Give your child another card with an arrow on it and have him or her match it to the other arrows.

Developing visual memory: Visual memory is the ability to reproduce letters or other objects and images from memory.

• Have your child circle all the words in a newspaper column that begin with a certain letter.

• Play "What's Missing?" Set out a few articles of clothing, for example. Have your child close her eyes while you remove one article. Have her tell which article is missing.

• Touch several objects on a table. Have your child try to touch the same objects, in the same order.

Eye Openers

- Alert, wide-open eyes are a good indicator of a healthy newborn baby.

- Ten percent of American children under twelve need vision correction. Six to ten million pairs of eyeglasses were dispensed to American children in 1989.

- Twenty-seven million Americans under the age of seventeen cannot read or write well enough to function in society. Another forty-five million are only marginally competent in these skills.

- Among children with learning disabilities, only 10 percent have a significant problem with their visual acuity. However, about 96 percent have focusing problems.

- The amount of light you need to comfortably watch TV in a room is about half the amount of light you need to read comfortably in the room.

- Arrange three shapes in a certain sequence. Mix them up and have your child arrange them in the same sequence.

- Open a story book to a certain page. Let your child look at it for a moment, and then close the book. See if your child can find the same page again.

- Write three numbers and quickly cover them. Ask your child to write what was seen.

Developing reading skills: For older children who have begun to read, here are some activities to do to encourage their abilities.

- Correct a mistake when your child is reading to you and misses a word, and have the child go right on so he or she does not lose concentration.

- Ask questions about what your child has read after he reads a page.

- Have your child look for words on a page that start or end with the same letter.

• Have your child look at the picture in a story. Have her guess what the story is about before reading it.

• Encourage your child to write his own stories.

• Let your child see you reading often. Imitation is a strong teacher.

For most children, vision, like other skills, develops on schedule with few problems. But, for some children, it does not, and it falls to the child's parents or teachers to pick up clues that vision or visual-motor skills may be lacking and to get the child the help he or she needs.

CHAPTER 5
How Your Eyes Age

Aging is one process that seems to be here to stay. True, some people put it off longer than others, but it eventually manages to catch up with each one of us. Every part of our body shows its age sooner or later, and the eyes are no exception. Researchers are continually trying to determine the cause for these changes and how they might be slowed or stopped. Some alternative methods of health care have shown some success in slowing down the aging process somewhat. Let's see exactly what happens to your eyes in those golden years.

Normal Age-Related Changes

Considering that they are probably among the most active, along with most exposed, parts of our body, it's no wonder the eyes go through some changes as your body ages. Some of these changes are normal and expected, while others can be dangerous and require prompt attention.

PRESBYOPIA—OR, YOUR SHORT ARMS

This book is about eyes, so why talk about short arms? Many of you who are over forty will know exactly why! During the first thirty to forty years of your life, your eyes have been busily working to see everything they could, especially reading and other near-point work. When your eyes are relaxed they are, theoretically, in focus for distant objects. When an object moves closer, you must actively focus the lens inside your eye to keep the object clear. This ability is very easy to do when we are young, but the maximum focusing ability is achieved when we are about five years old. As we get older, the eye's lens becomes stiffer, and the maximum focusing ability of the eye—actually the ability of the lens to become rounded as it must for near work—diminishes. Eventually, we notice a blur at close range.

Although this process of hardening of the lens is occurring constantly throughout our lifetime, it isn't given a name until we are unable to clear the near image comfortably. The condition is called *presbyopia* (prez-bee-OH-pee-ah); the word comes from the Greek word "presbys," which means "old."

Looking at this problem in persepctive should help give you a better idea of why this happens. Consider prehistoric man. In those early caveman days, the life expectancy was only about thirty to thirty-five years. The only near-point duties were maybe cooking and making weapons, neither of which is extremely detailed work. Most visual requirements at that time were distance tasks, like spotting that night's dinner, or keeping from becoming someone else's dinner. So really, our eyes were made to focus for our entire lifetime—except that we now outlive our eyes' focusing lifetime.

Treating Presbyopia

You can overcome presbyopia with a simple lens correction for near vision—in other words, reading glasses—or you can try a natural approach to slow the hardening of your eye's lenses. Of course, you might want to do both.

Corrective lenses: One way to compensate for the deficiency in the near vision is to get a prescription lens to help the eye with the focusing that it is unable to do anymore. If you already wear glasses to see clearly at a distance, then you'll need two different lens prescriptions, one for distance and one for near vision. One way to handle this double prescription is with *bifocals*, eyeglass lenses where the top lens is for distance vision and the lower lens for near work. Don't use the kind of reading glasses you can buy without a prescription in stores. They're not likely to be the exact prescription you need, and the lenses are of poor optical quality.

The natural approach: There is a school of thought that says that presbyopia is not an inevitable consequence of aging but is instead the result of years of improper nutrition, stress, improper exercise and lack of adequate oxygenation of the body. Even if you do everything right, you can't entirely prevent the development of presbyopia, but you may be able to postpone or slow down the hardening of the lens with good nutrition, aerobic exercise and generally healthful living. In my experience as an optometrist with the United States Navy, I noticed that the men who were in better shape had better vision for longer than those who were less fit. Like any part of the body, the lens will stay "younger" longer with the advantage of good overall health. In addition to general exercise and good nutrition, I recommend that patients who are reaching the "bifocal age" start doing a simple exercise several times a day. All you have to do is practice focusing from near to far (at least twenty feet away) and back to near again. This keeps the muscle that controls the lens in good working order. You can also try the accommodation exercises in chapter 9 (see *Accommodative Rock*, page 153 and *Deep Blink*, page 157).

PUPILS GET SMALLER

As people age, their pupils get slightly smaller. This phenomenon may occur because it's easier for the eyes to focus through a smaller pupil. More of the light going through a smaller hole will focus at a single point. In the eye, that point is your macula, the area of the retina that gives you the sharpest vision.

If you have presbyopia, hold some reading material near your eyes so that it looks blurry. Then try looking at the same material at the same distance but through a pinhole in a piece of paper. You'll find you can read the letters. If you're nearsighted, take off your glasses and get a blurry look at the world. Then look through your pinhole; the world should look a lot clearer through it. Looking through a pinhole gives you the same effect as looking through a smaller pupil. So, it's quite possible that the presbyopic eye is trying to compensate for its decreased flexibility in focusing by decreasing its pupil size. In any case, smaller pupils as we age are nothing to worry about.

A LIGHTER IRIS

There is also a tendency for the iris of our eyes to lighten slightly with age. This is due to a slight breakdown of the pigmented cells that are deposited in our irises. Although a dark brown eye won't turn bright blue, some graying in the iris can lighten the color of an older person's eyes. This doesn't really cause any problems except perhaps a slightly increased sensitivity to light. In fact, some people find it rather attractive.

SAGGING EYELIDS

The skin of your eyelids is very thin because it is designed to do much stretching. This constant movement can cause the upper lid skin to sag somewhat. There is usually no problem with this unless it sags far enough to interfere with the vision. A cosmetic surgery procedure called *blepharoplasty* (BLEF-er-oh-plas-tee) can take care of this problem. Consult an ophthalmologist or plastic surgeon who has had experience with this procedure.

Special Problems

Some problems associated with aging pose a real threat to your vision. Fortunately, many of them can now be treated.

CATARACTS

A word that strikes terror in the hearts of millions: *cataracts!* Stories have been passed down about people having their vision slowly fade into total blindness. But, most people don't know what a cataract is or why it represents a threat to vision.

What Is a Cataract?

A *cataract* is a clouding of the lens of the eye (*see* illustration, page 85). This clouding can be partial or complete, so not all cataracts interfere very much with vision. However, the type of cataract that occurs with advancing age is generally progressive,

Cataract

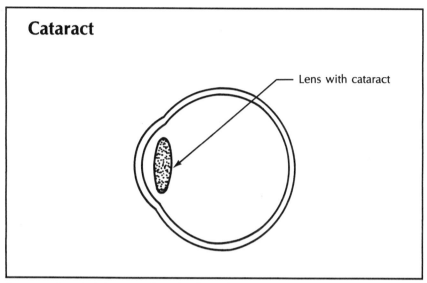

Lens with cataract

A cataract is a partial or complete clouding of the eye's lens, resulting in a diminution of vision in the eye. The most common type of cataract is the type that is associated with aging.

so that a small cataract that doesn't cause much of a problem will probably become a large cataract that obscures vision at some point, perhaps a few years down the road.

Cataracts are not limited to the aged, although so-called *senile cataracts* are the most common type of cataract. (No, having a senile cataract doesn't mean you're senile—that's just the medical way of saying "old.") Between the ages of sixty-five and seventy-four, about 23 percent of the population can be expected to have a cataract. After the age of seventy-five, about 50 percent of people will have one.

You may have heard that cataracts can also be present at birth. They can be, though it's pretty rare. They're called *congenital* and are sometimes caused by the mother's having contracted German measles, mumps, chickenpox or certain other infectious diseases during her pregnancy; they can also be inherited.

Some diseases, injuries and a class of anti-inflammatory drugs called *steroids* can also cause cataracts at any time of life. You can also develop a cataract after being exposed to radiation (from many X rays, for example), from constant exposure to infrared light (called "glassblower's cataract" because this profession used to work with infrared light without eye protection) or from being hit with a high-voltage current (lightning or electrocution) through the head. (Of course, if you're struck by lightning or electrocuted, cataracts would probably be the least of your concerns!) Recent research suggests that many years of exposure to ultraviolet light, which is part of sunlight but is beyond the human visible spectrum, can also play a part in the development of cataracts. Another new study suggests that cigarette smoking may be linked to the formation of cataracts; the eye damage seems to be from the effect of certain chemicals being transported internally to the lens when the person smokes, not from smoke in the environment.

Aging or Environment?

So, you may wonder, are cataracts an inevitable consequence of advancing age, or are they the result of something I'm doing that can be changed?

Researchers in the field of aging are asking this question about many conditions previously thought to be the unavoidable price of living a long life. The answer with cataracts, as with most conditions, is that they are probably a combination of the aging process and the environment in which the person has been living for many years. Years of exposure to ultraviolet light, radiation and various environmental "insults," such as smoking, eventually catch up with us as we age; at the same time, the eye's lens fibers begin to break down and are more vulnerable to stresses from the outside world. You may be able to prevent or postpone the development of a cataract by protecting your eyes against ultraviolet light with a good pair of sunglasses (see *Sunglasses*, page 116), eating a nutritious diet, limiting your exposure to infrared light and radiation from X rays and other sources, and by not smoking.

Living with a Cataract

If you do develop a cataract, you won't necessarily need surgery, at least not right away. What you'll notice with your cataract is that light is refracted differently now and doesn't look the same as it did before. You may see just a general sort of cloudy haze in your visual field, or you may see a "dazzling" effect of scattered light as it bounces off your cataract. Changes in how you see are almost always due to changes in the lighting around you.

Outdoors on a sunny day, you will probably want to wear a hat with a brim to reduce this "dazzle" effect of bright sunlight; sunglasses will help this too. Indoors, experiment with the best lighting for you. You'll find reading easier if you have a small reading lamp that can be moved around and adjusted for your comfort instead of a bright, immovable ceiling fixture. You may want to keep the room lighting low when you watch television.

Cataract Surgery

When the cataract is interfering significantly with your vision and your life, it's usually time to consider surgery (not every cataract gets to this point). You may have heard that you have to wait until a cataract is "ripe" before it can be surgically removed. This was true years ago, but new surgical techniques have made it possible to remove a cataract at any time as long as your doctor feels you are in good enough shape to undergo surgery. A few different surgical techniques can be used, and you and your surgeon can decide which one is best for you. Sometimes, cataract surgery can be done as an outpatient procedure.

Extracapsular cataract extraction: The eye's lens is surrounded by a capsule, which supports it in place. In this operation, only a bit of this capsule is removed, and the cataract-covered lens is either taken out or washed out of the capsule. The main advantage to this procedure is that most of the capsule stays in the eye to perform its function of dividing the front and back part of the eye and to support an artificial lens that can then be implanted in your eye (see *How You See After Cataract Removal*, page 88). Extracapsular extraction is now used about 65 percent of the time in cataract operations.

Intracapsular cataract extraction: Another way to remove a cataract is to remove the cataract-covered lens in its capsule; both the lens and lens capsule are removed. These days, the lens and capsule are usually frozen first to make extraction easier and to minimize bleeding. The main advantage of this method is that every bit of lens tissue and capsule tissue is removed so that no future cataract or cloudiness can form there. When the capsule is left in the eye, it may itself become opaque, or remnants of the old lens may grow over it and make it cloudy. These problems are known as *secondary cataract* or *aftercataract*. The main disadvantage is that, once the lens capsule is gone, the vitreous humor (remember, that's the gel in the back part of the eye) no longer has a "dam" to prevent its oozing into the front part of the eye, where it doesn't belong and can cause some trouble; there is also the problem of the capsule not being there to support an artificial lens implant.

Phacoemulsification: This technique (pronounced fack-oh-ee-MUL-si-fi-kay-shun and derived from the Greek word "phakos," which means lens) can be used during an extracapsular extraction. The cataract is broken up (made into an emulsion) using ultrasonic energy; it is then aspirated (sucked out). It has the advantage of a smaller incision and faster wound healing after surgery than other methods of extraction.

Contrary to what many people believe, lasers are not normally used in cataract surgery. Lasers burn holes in tissue, and a lens with a hole in it wouldn't do you any more good than a lens with a cataract. However, lasers are sometimes used in getting rid of a secondary cataract that has developed on the lens capsule after cataract surgery.

New and better procedures are now being developed to remove cataracts. The new procedures require smaller incisions and fewer complications (see *New Cataract Surgeries*, page 261).

How You See After Cataract Removal

By now you may be wondering: But, if my lens is removed, how do I see? Without a lens, you have very poor visual acuity. Fortunately, there are ways to get around this problem.

You may have heard of or seen people with "cataract glasses." Years ago, these heavy, thick glasses had to be worn after cataract surgery. They were not only unsightly, but they left something to be desired in terms of optical correction as well.

Nowadays, people who've had a lens removed replace it with either a contact lens worn on the cornea or with a plastic lens inserted into the eye during surgery right where their own lens used to be (it's called an artificial intraocular lens).

All of these solutions work for distance vision, but no artificial lens yet available can change shape to change your focus, although some are now in the early stages of research and development (see *New Cataract Surgeries*, page 261). Nor does changing the shape of the cornea give you the flexibility in focusing you need for both distance and near vision. So, in order to do near work like reading, you'll still need a glasses prescription—but so will most people your age!

GLAUCOMA

Glaucoma is a deceptive and dangerous eye disease. I say this because most glaucoma sufferers have few or no symptoms of the disease, which occurs in 1 to 2 percent of the over-forty population; yet, glaucoma is the second most common cause of blindness in the United States. A family history of glaucoma, diabetes, a previous eye injury or surgery, and the use of eye drops containing steroids are considered risk factors for developing glaucoma. It is also much more common in African-Americans than in white Americans.

What Is Glaucoma?

Glaucoma is a condition in which pressure inside the eye (intraocular pressure) is markedly elevated, which prevents blood from reaching and nourishing the eye and circulating through the eye.

In the normal eye, the aqueous humor is produced and drained from the eye (into the bloodstream) at a constant rate so that you always have a fresh supply and always the right amount of this fluid. The drainage takes place through a little canal between the iris and the cornea in each eye (*see* illustration, page 36 for a quick check on the anatomy here). In glaucoma, though, something goes wrong. Either too much aqueous humor is produced and the eye can't get rid of it fast enough to maintain normal intraocular pressure, or the drainage mechanism breaks down so that fluid can't escape fast enough to keep the pressure down to normal levels. Either way, the increased pressure interferes with blood circulation to and from the eye. The result is damage to the optic nerve with increasing loss of vision, peripheral vision being the first to go.

Sometimes there is an actual blockage of the drainage channel that a doctor can see. This type of glaucoma is called *narrow-angle* or *closed-angle* glaucoma. But, often the channel appears to be normal despite the elevated pressure. This is called *open-angle* glaucoma.

Glaucoma usually affects both eyes (unless it is caused by a specific injury or tumor in one eye), but the two eyes may not develop it at the same rate.

Detecting Glaucoma

About 15 percent of glaucoma patients know they have a problem. They have an acute form of glaucoma characterized by extreme eye pain, red eyes, dilated pupils, blurred vision and halos around lights in their vision. These people are lucky because they usually get themselves to an eye doctor promptly.

For the other 85 percent of glaucoma patients, the disease is chronic and insidious. The symptoms are subtle and may not even be noticed until a significant amount of vision has been lost. Contrary to popular conception, there is no feeling of pressure in the eye in the chronic type of glaucoma.

Fortunately, it's very easy for an optometrist or ophthalmologist to check for glaucoma by doing a simple test in his or her office to check for increased intraocular pressure. The most common test done today is the one where a puff of air is blown at your eye with a machine. Be sure you have this done every time you go in for a checkup. Another indication of glaucoma is a change in your peripheral vision and an enlarging blind spot. Unfortunately, people rarely notice such changes early on; they are detected when an eye doctor examines you. Your eye doctor should be checking these indicators regularly.

Is Aging the Cause?

As with most conditions, there is no single cause of glaucoma. We suspect that the general stiffening of the sclera and other parts of the eye plays a role in the development of glaucoma in people over forty. Other causes are serious eye injuries, eye surgeries, some medications (steroids are the main culprit here again) and tumors of the eye, to name a few. When children develop glaucoma during the first year of life, it is almost always due to an inherited malformation of the canal where the aqueous humor is supposed to drain.

Treating Glaucoma

Glaucoma can be treated medically (that is, with medications) or surgically, or both. The medical treatment involves the use of one or more of the following: eye drops to constrict the pupils (a constricted pupil opens the angle between the cornea and the iris to increase drainage of aqueous fluid); eye drops that reduce the production of aqueous fluid in the eye; and systemic medications that reduce the formation of aqueous fluid.

Some surgeries for glaucoma involve the creation of new channels from which the aqueous fluid can escape. In another procedure, a laser is used to burn little spots into the area around the iris. As these burns heal, they form scars and pull the tissue in toward them. This contracting of the tissue around the burns opens up the meshwork of the eye and reduces the overall intraocular pressure by increasing the drainage of aqueous fluid. Other procedures for glaucoma are now being developed (see *New Treatment for Glaucoma*, page 260).

MACULAR DEGENERATION

As you may remember from chapter 1, the macula is the area of the retina that is the most sensitive and is used for direct, central vision (reading, for example). For one in four people over the age of sixty-five and one in three over the age of eighty, the macula begins to degenerate (deteriorate).

Very often the macular area of one eye shows this degenerative change while the other eye is perfectly normal. In this circumstance, you may not notice that the change is taking place because the good eye will dominate.

Total blindness doesn't occur with macular degeneration. Since the macular area is only responsible for central vision, only this area will be affected. Peripheral vision usually remains intact and therefore allows a person to function almost normally, especially if only one eye is involved. Special low-vision aids can also be of great help to those with macular degeneration (see *Living with Low Vision*, page 92 and *New Vision Devices*, page 262).

What Causes Macular Degeneration?

The macula gets its nutrition from blood vessels in the choroid, so any condition that restricts blood flow over a long period of time can damage it. It is possible that *atherosclerosis* (ath-er-oh-skler-OH-sis), the clogging of the body's arteries with fatty plaques, is a contributor to the problem and a reason for it to occur in the later years. High blood pressure, diabetes, cigarette smoking, obesity, a diet high in fat and cholesterol and the genes we inherit from our parents can all contribute to atherosclerosis, and therefore to macular degeneration.

Preventing Macular Degeneration

Anything that prevents the clogging of your arteries may help prevent macular degeneration (as well as the degeneration of the rest of your body). Therefore, watching your dietary fat and cholesterol, exercising regularly, not smoking and watching your weight and blood pressure are wise moves. You can't do anything about your genes.

Some doctors are experimenting with having their older patients take zinc supplements to prevent or halt the progress of macular degeneration. In a study done at the Louisiana State University Eye Center, older adults who took zinc supplements for up to two years had less eye deterioration than people who didn't receive the supplements. But, since taking zinc can have serious side effects, including anemia and worsening of cardiovascular disease, don't run out to the health-food store and start dosing yourself with unlimited quantities of the stuff. Zinc should be taken under the supervision of a physician.

Treating Macular Degeneration

Lasers have been used in the treatment of one form of macular degeneration that is found in about 10 percent of cases. In this kind of macular degeneration, new blood vessels have sprouted in the wrong places, and the laser can be used to coagulate these vessels. Unfortunately, most forms of the problem cannot yet be reliably treated either medically or surgically.

LIVING WITH LOW VISION

Macular degeneration and other serious eye conditions in the later years can cause a decrease in vision that is not correctable with surgery, medication or ordinary optical lenses.

In recent years, some doctors and eye clinics have begun to specialize in patients who have low (also called "subnormal") vision and to provide these patients with high-tech solutions to their problem. (For the name of a doctor or clinic in your area, contact your local Optometric Society. The phone number should be listed in the yellow pages under "Optometrists." Also see the list of *Additional Resources* on page 266.)

For near vision, a simple magnifying glass can be of great help to you. You can also get magnifying glasses with lights attached and some that go around your neck so you can look through them without using your hands while reading or sewing.

Extremely high magnification of printed material can be obtained with closed-circuit television. The print is held under the television camera, magnified and shown on a television screen. For the truly blind, print can actually be "read" by a small camera and then converted into a pattern that can be felt with

Eye Openers

• The onset of presbyopia is one of the first signs of an aging body. There are now twenty-seven million "presbyopes" in the United States who need glasses for reading.

• In 1987, thirty-two million pairs of bifocals were dispensed in the United States.

• A white ring around the eye's cornea, which was previously thought to be a normal sign of aging, has now been associated with a high level of blood cholesterol and an increased risk of heart disease, according to a study released by the American Optometric Association in 1990. Optometrists recommend that if you have such a ring, you should have your blood cholesterol level checked by your doctor.

• Forty-one million Americans over the age of forty have age-related cataracts, and four hundred thousand new cataracts develop each year.

• Cataract surgery is the most common surgery done in the United States today. Its cost is over $1.5 billion. Forty-three percent of all surgeries performed in the United States are for cataracts.

• In a study released in 1990, it was found that of 838 Maryland fishermen between the ages of thirty and ninety-four, those who smoked were twice as likely to have developed a cataract prior to age seventy than those who had quit smoking at least ten years previously. The study suggests that damage to the eye's lens may be reversible if the person stops smoking.

• About two million Americans have glaucoma; over nine hundred thousand of these suffer a permanent loss of vision, and about seventy thousand are made blind by the disease.

• Over eleven million people in the United States suffer from visual impairment that cannot be corrected with eyeglasses or contact lenses. Of these, 0.5 million are legally blind, and 1.5 million are so severely impaired that they cannot read ordinary newsprint.

your finger. Of course, this type of equipment is expensive, but it may be worth it if it enables you to keep earning a living or doing what you like to do.

For distance vision, small telescopes, which can be adjusted for focus, can be attached to your glasses. They greatly restrict your field of vision, but they may make it possible for you to see clearly within the smaller field. Pocket telescopes are also available for use in reading such things as street signs and bus numbers.

A positive attitude and a little ingenuity can go a long way in adapting to low vision. Put a raised dot on your oven at 350 degrees; learn to dial or punch the numbers on your phone without having to look; feel the edges of papers and learn how to sign your name on a straight line without looking. Get involved in a regular exercise program, keep good music and books on tape at hand, and seek out the large-print book collection at your local library. Many communities offer support groups for those with low vision that can help you with the emotional and practical aspects of your condition.

Not all changes that happen with age are bad. Advertisers tell us that we should spend our money trying to look the same year after year and that aging is ugly. Of course, we do change with age, and that's not all bad. After all, maturation does have some advantages. Gray hair, sagging eyelids and even a cataract or two may be the price we have to pay to obtain it. Fortunately, there are now surgeries and nonsurgical treatments available for more and more of the serious problems that sometimes accompany aging.

CHAPTER 6
Finding Eye Care

What's the difference between an ophthalmologist, an optometrist and an optician? Talk about confusing! In studies done time and time again it is found that the public still gets these professions confused and probably always will.

OPHTHALMOLOGISTS, OPTOMETRISTS, OPTICIANS

Let's see if I can set you straight on the three types of eye-care professionals.

Opththalmologists: An *ophthalmologist* (of-thal-MAHL-oh-jist) is a medical doctor (M.D.) who specializes in eye health and disease. After he or she graduates from college and medical school, an ophthalmologist spends three more years learning about diseases and surgeries of the eye (all ophthalmologists are surgeons). In order to be what is known as a "board-certified" ophthalmologist, the M.D. must pass a written, oral and practical certifying exam in the specialty of ophthalmology. He or she must then either take fifteen hours of continuing education per year or a hundred hours every four years.

So, as you can see, an ophthalmologist has a lot of training. But, that doesn't mean an ophthalmologist is the right professional for every eye problem. Ophthalmologists are the people to see with eye diseases requiring medications or surgery and when you have a serious eye injury.

Most ophthalmologists prescribe glasses and contact lenses for healthy eyes, but many refer all or part of this type of work to someone else. For example, in a recent survey of about six hundred ophthalmologists, 75 percent indicated that someone in their practices fitted contact lenses, but only 60 percent did the fitting themselves (the rest had technicians or optometrists do it).

Ophthalmologists sometimes subspecialize within the specialty of ophthalmology. Some are *retinologists,* specializing in problems of the retina. Others specialize in problems of the cornea, iris or lens. Some are pediatric ophthalmologists, specializing in children's eye problems. Some confine themselves to surgery or to specific kinds of surgery, such as surgery for cataracts.

Optometrists: An *optometrist* (op-TAHM-e-trist) is a doctor of optometry (O.D.). Optometrists are "doctors," but they are not "medical doctors" (M.D.'s). After graduating from college, an optometrist goes to a four-year school of optometry, where he or she learns all the different aspects of vision and visual perception, as well as how to recognize eye diseases and serious injuries. The optometrist works with healthy eyes that cannot function properly. If the optometrist suspects eye disease or a serious injury, he or she normally refers the patient to an ophthalmologist for treatment. (In some states optometrists are allowed to treat certain eye diseases and injuries.)

Optometrists must be licensed in each state. There is a national board exam for licensing in optometry, and most states accept passage of the national exam along with an additional practical or oral exam of their own.

Optometrists also have their areas of specialization. Some of these are: contact lenses; low vision (see *Living with Low Vision,* page 92); vision therapy (see *Vision Therapy,* page 149); sports vision (*see* chapter 11); industrial vision (*see* chapter 10); and the subspecialty *orthokeratology,* which involves using contact lenses to change the shape of the cornea to correct a vision problem (see *Reshaping the Cornea with Contact Lenses,* page 143).

The best way to find a contact lens specialist may be to find a friend who has had a good experience with his or her contacts. Some optometrists restrict their practices to contact lenses, but that in itself is not a reason to choose one of them for your contact lens needs.

There is now a College of Optometrists in Vision Development and an International Orthokeratology Society to educate specialists in vision therapy and in orthokeratology, respectively (*see* the list of *Additional Resources* on page 266). Your local or county Optometric Society can also refer you to these optometric specialists and to other optometric specialists in your area (check your phone directory under "Optometrists" to get to your Optometric Society).

Opticians: An *optician* (op-TISH-an) is a technician who is trained to fill prescriptions for lenses written by optometrists or ophthalmologists. They are trained to make glasses, fit eyeglass lenses into frames and adjust glasses frames to a person's face. In some states, opticians are allowed to do the fitting of contact lenses.

The usual course for opticians is an associate college degree, which is normally a two-year program. Most states license opticians and require continuing education. There is an American Board of Opticianry, which certifies opticians; this certification may or may not be accepted by a particular state as qualifying an optician to practice. At this time, requirements vary a great deal from state to state.

All three of these professionals have an important job to do in maintaining your visual well-being. The best way to know who to see is to read this book carefully and become familiar with your eyes so you know what to do and who to go to for help.

ASK QUESTIONS

OK, so now you know what kind of professional you want. But, how do you know whether you've got the right person? This is a tough one! There are as many types of professionals as there are types of people. One of the best sources of good doctors is word of mouth. If you have a friend who wears glasses or contacts and has been with a good doctor for years, there's a good chance that will be a good doctor for you.

Don't be too sold on young professionals who are fresh out of school. Although they may have the latest technical knowledge, there's something to be said for experience in any profession. And, some new doctors are so cautious that they may keep you in the chair for hours doing every test in the book instead of just the ones that relate to your problem.

To avoid the high costs of setting up an office of their own, new graduates of optometry school will sometimes begin their practices in chain-store operations, which are usually located in shopping malls. In these kinds of stores, you will often see a young doctor with good technical knowledge but little time to apply it because of the large number of patients the store books into each time slot.

On the other hand, be cautious of the older doctor who has been in the same location since prehistoric times. Many of them are fine if they have kept up with the advancements in eye-care technology and knowledge, but things are changing fast and not everyone keeps up. Since most states require continuing education as part of the relicensing process for optometrists, checking to make sure that your doctor has a valid license should give you some comfort that he or she has kept abreast of at least the most important developments in the field.

I don't advise browsing through the yellow pages for a doctor. It still amazes me how many people will choose an eye doctor simply based on who has the biggest ad or on how much the exam costs. Do they also shop around for bargain-priced brain surgeons?

Here are a few questions to ask the receptionist when you first call for an appointment:

- How long has the doctor been in practice?

- How long does the examination take?

- Will my eyes be dilated for the examination?

- How much does the examination cost?

- How long has that particular office been open?

Here are some questions to ask the doctor before he or she starts the examination:

- Do you take a case history? (Be sure the doctor sits down and talks about your problems, medical history, medications and lifestyle.)

- How extensive is your examination form? (Although it will probably look mysterious, see how big it is and how much of it gets filled up when the examination is complete. Be suspicious of an examination form that's the size of an index card.)

- Do you perform a full range of distance and near tests?

• Is a glaucoma test a regular part of the examination?

• Do you work with a number of different contact lens companies? (It's important if you want contact lenses to have a doctor who is not tied to one product for every eye. There are many different kinds of contact lenses out there now.)

• Do you describe the different tests as you perform them?

• Do you offer alternatives in treatment according to patient preference, such as contacts, glasses or vision therapy?

• Do you regularly refer to other doctors for medical conditions that you recognize or for special kinds of treatments and therapies that you don't offer?

Much of what you determine will be based on just plain old gut feelings about the office in general. If you feel you aren't getting high-quality, personalized service from your eye doctor, you may want to go elsewhere. Sometimes it takes a little faith and trust to find a good eye-care professional. A good doctor is hard to find, but once you find one, stay with him or her and appreciate the good vision care.

WHAT IS AN EYE EXAM?

A complete eye examination should be so thorough that it tires you out! Here are some basic areas that should be included in a complete eye exam.

Case history: Your doctor should ask you questions starting with: "Why are you here?" He or she should ask you about the date of your last examination, your history of glasses or contact lenses, the quality of your distance and near vision, any headaches you may be having, any medications you may be taking, your job-related visual tasks and any family history of eye diseases. Beware of a doctor who doesn't ask you any questions before beginning his or her work!

Visual acuity testing: This means testing the sharpness of your vision using the Snellen chart. Each eye is tested individually for distance and then again for near. This will give the doctor an idea of how well you see the world.

External eye health: The doctor should check the outer areas of the eye, including the pupil, iris, cornea, sclera, conjunctiva, lids, eyelashes, eyebrows and the skin area surrounding the eyes. This is usually done with a flashlight, although occasionally more sophisticated instruments that magnify the eye are used.

Ophthalmoscope exam: Using an *ophthalmoscope* (of-THAL-moh-scope), the doctor will look into the back of your eye to see the retina, optic nerve, blood vessels and surrounding tissue to rule out any diseases in those areas.

Refraction: Used in this sense, refraction means the determination of refractive errors (see *Nearsighted or Farsighted?*, page 22) in your vision. This is done when you look through the machine called a *refractor* that contains all the lens combinations (*see* illustration, page 101). Using this instrument, the doctor can determine your distance prescription and near prescription. The refractor also gives information about your eye-muscle balance, focusing strength and focusing flexibility. This portion of the exam will probably be the longest.

Glaucoma testing: A normal part of the eye exam for adults consists of a glaucoma test. The pressure of the eye is measured with an instrument called a *tonometer* (*see* illustration, page 102). Most of today's tonometers are of the type that blow a puff of air at the eye. Although this can be the most irritating part of the exam, it is also the most crucial.

Visual field testing: The doctor may perform a visual field examination to determine whether your peripheral vision is intact. This is most often done if glaucoma is suspected, but it can be done at any time, and some doctors do it routinely. The old-fashioned way to test visual fields was with a black felt board and a white-tipped pointer; the patient indicated to the doctor the time at which he or she could see the pointer in his peripheral vision. Modern visual field testing is done using a computerized system. The patient's head is put into a shell-like contraption and lights are flashed around his head. The patient indicates when he sees these flashes.

Other tests: There are many other areas that the doctor can investigate, depending on your particular needs. For example, contact lens fitting will require a measurement of the curvature of the cornea.

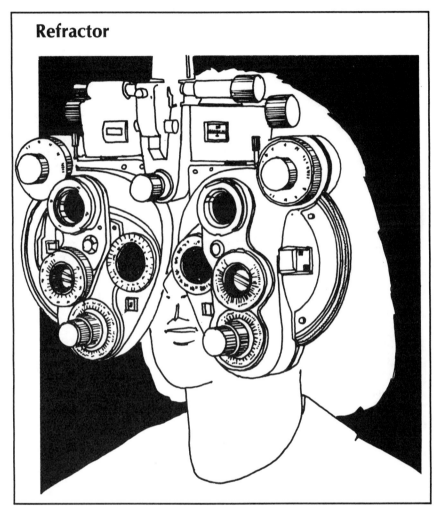

Refractor

An eye doctor can determine your degree of refractive error and your corrective lens prescription by using an instrument called a refractor, which contains all possible lens combinations. This instrument also gives a doctor some information about your eye-muscle balance and the focusing mechanism of each eye.

Dilated exam: Many patients wonder whether eye drops that dilate (widen) the pupil will be used during an eye examination and how long the drops take to wear off. Drops are sometimes used for either of two purposes: to enable the doctor to get a better view of the inner eye for detection of eye diseases and retinal problems; and to paralyze the focusing muscle of the eye. Some doctors dilate eyes routinely, but if the exam room is dark, the

Tonometer

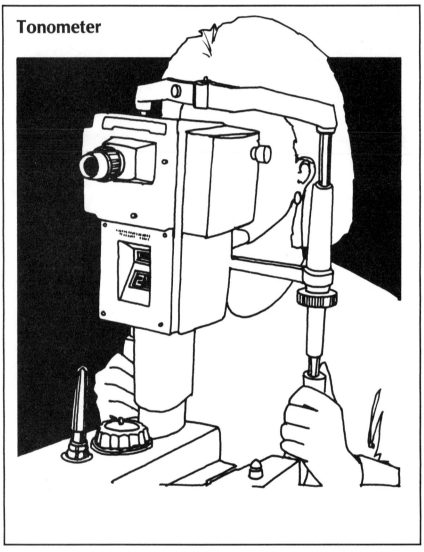

The tonometer measures pressure inside the eye and screens patients for glaucoma (a disease involving elevated eye pressure). Modern tonometers work by blowing a puff of air at the eye.

pupils of most patients are dilated enough so that the exam can be conducted without dilating drops. It may be necessary to use drops in older patients with very small pupils, especially if eye disease is suspected, and in children, where the drops may be used to paralyze the focusing muscle if the child is unable to

Eye Openers

• In 1988, 26.6 percent of Americans had their eyes examined.

• A 1989 survey of 448 consumers in the United States who had either had an eye exam in the last two years or had arranged for a household member to have one revealed a lot of misunderstanding about ophthalmologists and optometrists. Thirty-nine percent of the respondents said they understood the differences between ophthalmologists and optometrists. However, further questioning revealed that: 60 percent of those surveyed did not know that both may use drops to examine eyes; only 12 percent knew that neither grinds lenses for glasses; 68 percent were unaware that both kinds of professionals are graduates of four-year professional degree programs; only 60 percent knew that ophthalmologists held the M.D. degree; and 82 percent did not know that the services of both professions are covered by Medicare.

• In the United States in 1990, there were: 17,500 ophthalmologists, 30,000 optometrists and 27,000 opticians. Stated another way: For every ophthalmologist, there were 1.71 optometrists and 1.54 opticians.

focus at the required distances for the exam. Doctors may also use the drops if unusual refractive problems are suspected in a patient. A dilated eye will usually return to normal by the morning after the exam. In the meantime, the patient will be extremely sensitive to light and will be unable to read or focus for any near-point activities.

Consultation after the exam: Following the examination, the doctor should spend some time explaining the results and his or her recommendation for your eyes. Be certain that you understand the results of the testing and all the options that are given to you. Be cautious of a doctor who pushes one option.

COST OF AN EYE EXAM

It's difficult to put a price on eye care, but you should have some idea of what to expect when you want a complete eye exam. Prices for exams, contact lenses and other services vary in different parts of the country.

A survey of optometrists published in August 1989 found the national average cost for a complete exam including fitting for contact lenses (if desired by the patient) to be $48. A similar survey of ophthalmologists in 1988 found the average cost for a comprehensive exam was $58 with additional charges for contact lens fitting.

Sometimes you'll see "specials" on eye exams. These are popular in shopping malls and are designed to entice you into the store where, it is hoped, you will purchase other services, such as contact lenses or glasses. In other words, the exam is a "loss leader" and is part of a "bait-and-switch" technique used by some practitioners. I suggest that you stay away from them.

I don't think people should do much shopping around when it comes to their vision. Find a professional you can trust, and stick with him or her. Quality doesn't usually come cheap.

CHAPTER 7

Your Glasses

Most of us don't think very much about our glasses. But, the fact is, millions of us wouldn't be able to function without them. It's worth taking a look at how your glasses work, how they're made and how to find a pair that's both attractive and durable.

MINUS AND PLUS LENSES

There are two basic types of lenses that can be prescribed for vision correction: the *minus* lens, for correction of myopia, and the *plus* lens, for correction of hyperopia. These lenses are illustrated on page 106. You may also want to look at *Nearsighted or Farsighted?* on page 22 to refresh your memory on what happens in the nearsighted and farsighted eye.

The minus lens is concave in shape, thinner in the center than at the edges. Because of its shape, the minus lens *weakens* the focusing power of the light before it enters the eye, so that an image the eye is looking at falls *farther back*, onto the retina. The minus lens is needed for the nearsighted eye to see clearly.

The plus lens is a convex lens, much like the shape of the eye's own lens. It is thicker in the center than at the edges and *increases* the focusing power of light before it enters the eye. Images fall *farther forward* in relation to the retina when a convex lens is in front of the eye. This increase in focusing power is needed for the farsighted eye to see clearly.

You may remember from chapter 5 (see *Presbyopia*, page 81) that presbyopia is a normal part of aging; the eye's own lens hardens and can no longer accommodate to see things up close. A lens that moves images farther forward onto the retina (in

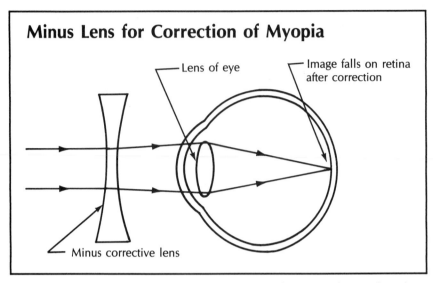

Minus Lens for Correction of Myopia

Lens of eye

Image falls on retina after correction

Minus corrective lens

The minus lens is concave in shape and thinner in the center than at the edges. Because of its shape, the minus lens weakens the focusing power of the light before it enters the eye, so that an image the eye is looking at falls farther back, onto the retina.

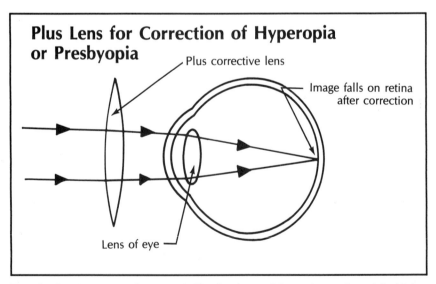

Plus Lens for Correction of Hyperopia or Presbyopia

Plus corrective lens

Image falls on retina after correction

Lens of eye

The plus lens is a convex lens, much like the shape of the eye's own lens. It is thicker in the center than at the edges and increases the focusing power of light before it enters the eye. Images fall farther forward in relation to the retina when a convex lens is in front of the eye.

other words, a lens that corrects hyperopia) can compensate for a lens that cannot accommodate for near vision. So, a plus lens is used to correct presbyopia as well as hyperopia.

Lenses for astigmatism are usually a combination of plus and minus lenses to fit the particular curvatures of the astigmatic eye.

Your lenses will not look like the ones in our illustration because of the way lenses are now manufactured, but the principle on which they work is the same.

Your optometrist will prescribe exactly the lens power you need. He or she will also measure the distance between the pupils of your eyes when they are focused for both distance and near vision and make sure the lenses' optical centers (the part you look through when you're looking straight ahead) correspond to that distance.

Beware of the do-it-yourself prescription reading glasses available in drugstores and discount stores. The lenses are not of high optical quality, and, needless to say, they are not made with your exact prescription in mind. The optical centers of the drugstore lenses will probably be different from those of your eyes, which can cause a lot of eyestrain. Also, do-it-yourself lenses can't compensate for astigmatism.

BIFOCALS

So, minus lenses correct for nearsightedness, and plus lenses correct for farsightedness and presbyopia. But, what do you do if you're already nearsighted and then become presbyopic as you get older (a common situation)? You'll still need your distance prescription to see the TV or the road when you're driving, but you'll find as you age that you'll also need some correction for very close work like reading. In other words, you now have a problem with *both* near and distance vision and have only a narrow range in between at which you can see without correction. You could keep wearing your distance glasses for getting around in the world and get a pair of reading glasses for near work, and some people do this. Or, you could enter the world of bifocals.

Bifocals, as the word implies, are lenses that have two focal corrections—one for near and one for distance. If your examination reveals a need for bifocals, take heart; you aren't the first and won't be the last. Let's take a look at bifocals and see where they came from and where they're going. You might be surprised.

The first bifocal was developed by Benjamin Franklin in the late 1700s. He took his distance glasses and cut them in half, then took his reading glasses and cut them in half and then glued the two halves together so the distance lens was on top of the near lens. This primitive but functional solution kept Franklin from having to switch back and forth between two pairs of glasses.

In 1908, John Borsch, Jr. created the first "fused" bifocal by cutting a segment out of the lower portion of a distance lens, inserting a glass material of higher density than the distance lens (for near vision) and then heating the two sections to melt them together. The lines were not as obvious as the Franklin bifocal, but the optics were not that sharp either.

The first good one-piece bifocal came along in 1910 when technology allowed for the production of a single glass lens with two different curves, one curve for each focal point. The reading segment was large, but the line between the segments was obvious, and the glass lenses were heavy. This is the same type of lens used even today in the "executive" bifocal with a line going all the way across the lens. They are now available in either glass or plastic. The major drawbacks are the prominent line between the segments and the "jump" of the image as the eye passes from distance to near.

The most popular type of bifocal in recent times has been the "flat-top" bifocal. The flat-top is similar to the fused lens invented by Borsch, but the top portion of the reading segment is made of the same material as the distance lens, so that when the lenses are fused, that material "disappears" and leaves a crescent reading segment. This lens has some significant optical advantages, as well as having a very thin, hardly noticeable line. Many of today's bifocals are made this same way.

In 1946, a bifocal was developed that was similar again to the Borsch lens, but the junction between the distance and near segments were blended to reveal no noticeable line. This was cosmetically appealing because no one could tell that the lens was a bifocal. However, when the wearer changed focus from distance to near and back, his vision blurred significantly in the transition zone between the two segments. This was unacceptable to most wearers. Even today, the "no-line" bifocals have not been a good solution for most people. "Flat-top" bifocals are what most wearers prefer.

TRIFOCALS AND PAL'S

Bifocals are adequate for most people with a need for both distance and near corrections; most people's eyes can focus for intermediate distances—such as computer work, card playing, music reading, seeing prices on grocery shelves and working on a large desk—either by using their distance lens segment or their near lens segment. But, there are some patients whose eyes also need a special lens for this intermediate, "arms-length" distance. The answer for this kind of problem is—you guessed it—*trifocals!* Trifocals correct vision at *three* different focal lengths.

The first trifocals were first developed in the 1940s and were of similar design to the flat-top segments we just discussed, except for having an additional segment between the reading and distance segments that was focused for an intermediate distance. The fitting of these lenses was extremely difficult. People needed the intermediate segment to be low enough so that they could comfortably look through the distance segment while driving but high enough so they could comfortably look through the reading segment in the grocery store—and they wanted to be able to keep their heads in a normal position for these activities! It was no surprise that few people adapted well to trifocals in the early days.

The next evolution came in the early 1950s in France, when Bernard Maitenaz developed a single lens that incorporated the distance, intermediate and reading prescriptions without any visible lines. The lens was called a *progressive addition lens (PAL)*, which meant that the power change from distance to near was gradual and uninterrupted—similar to the way the eye normally functions. Unfortunately, Maitenaz's first-generation design made for severe distortions at the edges of the lens, which created a "swimming" motion when the wearer walked.

These days, technological advances in optics have overcome most of the problems and have improved Maitenaz's lens so that it is now the correction of choice in many situations. There are now about twenty companies making progressive addition lenses, and the latest versions seem to be easy to adapt to and comfortable to wear. People who need an intermediate-distance correction use the central intermediate lens area with ease and no noticeable difficulty; they use the bottom part of the lens for very close work and the topmost area for distance. The head positions, although still a consideration, are not nearly as much a complicating factor because of the gradual transition in lens powers.

UNDERSTANDING YOUR EYEGLASS PRESCRIPTION

If you have ever had a prescription for glasses, you may have noticed that it looked rather confusing. What ever happened to 20/20? As you may remember from our earlier discussion about 20/20, a prescription for glasses cannot be derived from your reading letters on a chart. Look at the illustrations on pages 111 and 112, and I'll explain how to read a prescription so you can judge for yourself how your eyes are doing.

The basic prescription is broken down into two general categories: distance vision and near vision. In the illustrations on pages 111 and 112, you'll see the abbreviations "OD" and "OS." These stand for the Latin words for right eye—"oculus dexter"— and left eye—"oculus sinister." Some prescription forms today simply say "right" and "left" or "R" and "L."

The first column on the left—"SPHERE" in our illustrations— contains the basic lens power. If the numbers in this column are preceded by a minus sign, the prescription is for minus lenses that correct for nearsightedness. If the numbers are preceded by a plus sign, the prescription is for plus lenses to correct for farsightedness. (It is possible to be farsighted in one eye and nearsighted in the other, although this is uncommon.) The units of measurement are called *diopters*, a measurement of the refractive power of a lens. A larger number indicates more correction. A typical prescription for a mildly nearsighted patient would be about − .25 to − 1.50 diopters; − 1.75 to − 3.00 would be a moderate prescription; more than − 3.25 would be considered a significant myopia correction; and a − 6.00 or more would be a prescription for severe myopia. For farsightedness, up to about + 1.50 would be considered a mild prescription; + 1.50 to + 2.50 would be for moderate hyperopia; and over + 2.50 would be to correct significant hyperopia.

In the nearsighted prescription in the illustration on page 111, the patient needs a distance correction of − 1.00 in his right eye and − 2.25 in his left. (Quiz questions: Which eye is worse—the patient's left or right? Would his right eye be considered mildly, moderately or severely nearsighted? What about his left eye?)

In the prescription in the illustration on page 112, the patient is farsighted. Her right eye needs a distance correction of + 1.50 diopters and her left eye a correction of + 0.50 diopters. (Is she

Eyeglass Prescription
to Correct Nearsightedness

FOR ___MR. JOHN DOE___

EXAM
DATE _____

℞		SPHERE	CYLINDER	AXIS	PRISM	BASE
D I S T.	OD	−1.00	−0.75	180	—	—
	OS	−2.25	−1.25	75	—	—
N E A R	OD					
	OS					

PD ___64/60___ SPECIAL INSTRUCTIONS _____

_____ O.D.

"Minus" notations in the "SPHERE" column indicate a prescription for near-sightedness. This patient needs a correction of − 1.00 diopters in the right eye and − 2.25 diopters in the left eye. The patient also has some astigmatism, the correction for which is indicated in the "CYLINDER" and "AXIS" columns. The "PD" stands for "pupillary distance," and the fraction represents the distance between the pupils (in millimeters) when they are focused for distance over the distance between them when they are focused for near vision. The "PRISM" and "BASE" columns are for special conditions.

mildly, moderately or significantly farsighted in each eye?) A similar prescription might be written for a presbyopic patient.

The second and third columns for both prescriptions are "CYLINDER" and "AXIS"; they indicate the amount and the direction of any astigmatism you may have. Picture the normal eye as being shaped like a basketball (spherical) and the astigmatic eye more like a football (a squashed sphere). The CYLINDER column is for the amount of correction the astigmatic eye needs; it's expressed in diopters with a plus or minus sign. The *direction* of the astigmatism refers to which way the "football" is turned; it's expressed in degrees and is always between 1 and 180. The nearsighted patient whose prescription is illustrated has astigmatism in both eyes. The farsighted patient needs correction for astigmatism only in the left eye. Changes in near-sighted and farsighted prescriptions are common over time.

Eyeglass Prescription
to Correct Farsightedness

FOR Ms. JANE DOE   EXAM
DATE

℞		SPHERE	CYLINDER	AXIS	PRISM	BASE
D I S T.	OD	+1.50	—	—	—	—
	OS	+0.50	-0.50	90	—	—
N E A R	OD					
	OS					

PD _64/60_ SPECIAL INSTRUCTIONS _____

_____ O.D.

"Plus" notations in the "SPHERE" column indicate a prescription for farsightedness. This patient needs a correction of +1.50 diopters in the right eye and +0.50
in the left eye. The left eye has some astigmatism, as indicated in the "CYLINDER"
and "AXIS" column, but the right eye does not.

Astigmatism normally remains about the same once a person
reaches adulthood, although minor changes normally occur
after the sixth decade of life.

The next column on both prescriptions is headed "PRISM." A
prism correction bends light and may be prescribed for special
problems. It isn't very common. The final column—"BASE"—
refers to whether the base of the prism in the lens should be
pointing up, down, in or out.

The "PD" on the form is for the "pupillary distance"—the
distance between the patient's pupils. There are usually two
numbers, written as they are in these illustrations: 64/60. This
figure expresses the distance between your pupils at distance
over the distance between them at near. They are measured in
millimeters and don't change after you're fully grown.

Most states require that an eyeglass prescription expire at the
end of one year, although some allow it to go to two years. You
should be getting your eyes checked more often than that
anyway!

LENSES—GLASS? PLASTIC? COATED?

Up until the late 1950s, all glasses lenses were made out of glass (that's why they weren't called "eyeplastics"!). Since then, however, the advent of a newer optical plastic called *CR-39®* has revolutionized lenses. This material was originally developed during World War II and was further refined to improve its optical properties. A new kind of plastic lens, called a *polycarbonate* plastic lens, has now entered the market and has some advantages over the CR-39® lens.

CR-39® plastic is now used in about 80 percent of American lens prescriptions. This plastic's main advantage over glass is that it is light in weight—about 50 percent of the weight of glass lenses per diopter of power. This makes it much more comfortable to wear, especially in the higher prescriptions (whether they're for near—or farsightedness). Plastic is also much more protective for the eyes. Although it can still break, it takes a much greater force to break plastic lenses than glass ones, and plastic doesn't splinter into tiny slivers as glass does. The lenses can be tinted different colors easily (glass is not so easy to tint although it can be done), and the color can also be changed if desired. Plastic lenses can be treated to block out ultraviolet light (glass lenses block UV light without being treated), which makes it as good a material for sunglasses as glass is. If you like rimless frames, plastic is the lens of choice because it won't chip at the exposed edge nearly as easily as glass will.

In 1985 a new type of plastic lens—the *polycarbonate* plastic lens—was introduced. The "bending power" of this lens material is such that lenses can be thinner than the CR-39® plastic lenses and yet achieve equal optical power. This polycarbonate lens is also 50 percent lighter than conventional plastic, has inherent ultraviolet protection and can be treated to be scratch-resistant. One of the most impressive properties of this lens is that it is practically unbreakable. A twelve-gauge shotgun fired at the lens at close range only dented it! This is obviously the ideal lens to use in protective eyewear. The only drawback in using the lens is that the usable "optical zone" (the part you see through) is slightly narrower than that of a conventional plastic lens, so distortions in the wearer's peripheral vision can occur, which bothers some people with higher prescriptions.

The chief disadvantage of both CR-39® and polycarbonate plastics is that they scratch more easily than glass. Scratch-resistant coatings are now available that can be applied to the surface of a plastic lens to reduce its susceptibility to scratching. These are very effective and I recommend them, but they admittedly do not approximate the hardness of glass.

Glass lenses are still available and do have certain advantages. If you have a mild prescription and don't select a very large frame, their weight may not be a problem, and they are more scratch-resistant than plastic. The ability to block out ultraviolet light is inherent in glass lenses.

Glass lenses can be made as *photochromic* lenses, which means they can react to light and automatically darken as the surrounding light gets brighter, such as when you move from indoors to a sunny outdoor environment (see *What Color Lens?*, page 118). Plastic lenses are not yet available as photochromics. However, ordinary tinting does not work as well in glass as in plastic lenses. It can't be changed if you change your mind about the color, and it isn't as uniform in the higher prescriptions as it is with a plastic lens.

The main problem with glass lenses, in addition to their weight, is that they can splinter when broken and seriously injure your eyes. Today's glass lenses are tempered to minimize splintering (such tempering is now a federal law) but they are still not as safe as plastic lenses. I wouldn't wear them to play baseball.

So, which is the best lens for you? Well, if you just have to wear glasses occasionally for reading, and you have a tendency to toss them around carelessly, glass is the best way to go. If you wear glasses on a full-time basis, but your prescription is not very high, CR-39® plastic will do nicely. If your prescription is very high or you're in a high-risk environment for breakage, polycarbonate is for you. For kids, who are always tough on glasses, either glass or polycarbonate is recommended, depending on the prescription. Glass will certainly last longer and not scratch as badly, but polycarbonate is much safer. Ask your optician for his or her recommendations.

Lens Coatings

Have you ever noticed how in photographs of people wearing glasses you probably can see their glasses but not their eyes? That's because of the reflection of the room lights or sunlight off the front surface of their glasses. This occurs because only 92 percent of light passes through a lens, with 8 percent bouncing

Eyeglass Lenses

Lens Characteristics	Glass	CR-39® Plastic	Polycarbonate Plastic
Weight	Heavy	Light	Lightest
Impact Resistance	Fair	Good	Excellent
Tintability	Fair	Excellent	Good
UV Protection	Excellent (Inherent)	Can Be Treated	Excellent (Inherent)
Scratch Resistance	Excellent	Fair	Fair
Thickness per Diopter	Thick	Thicker	Thinnest
Availability as Photochromic Lens	Yes	No	No
Suitable for Rimless Frames	No	Yes*	Yes

*in lower prescriptions

off the surface of the eyeglass lenses. A new *anti-reflective* lens coating has recently been developed to take care of this problem. The coating has some distinct advantages. With an anti-reflective coating on the lens, 99 percent of the light can pass through the lens; only about 1 percent is deflected. An observer can see the wearer's eyes through these lenses and sometimes not perceive that the wearer is wearing lenses at all. Some people consider this a major cosmetic advantage, especially in the higher prescriptions, where rings of reflected light are occasionally visible in the lens. The wearer who drives at night will appreciate that the coating also eliminates glare from oncoming headlights. One disadvantage: Anti-reflective coatings tend to smudge and need special cleaning and handling.

Lenses can also be treated with coatings that block UV light, coatings for scratch resistance, mirror coatings (for sunglasses) and tinted coatings. The photochromic process is not a coating.

Coating your lenses may add twenty-five to fifty dollars to the price of your glasses (at 1990 prices).

Discuss different lens materials and coatings with your optometrist and optician. Find out what's available and which products best suit your needs.

SUNGLASSES

Sunglasses have traditionally been worn for style at any time and comfort in bright sunlight. Recent research has added protection from harmful light rays to the list of reasons to wear sunglasses. Any eyeglass prescription can be made in a tinted lens for use in sunlight. If you don't already wear glasses, you should get a pair of quality nonprescription sunglasses to protect your eyes.

Protection from Ultraviolet Light

As you learned in chapter 3, ultraviolet (UV) light—also called "ultraviolet radiation"—is light that is not visible to the human eye because it is below the visible spectrum in wavelength. (It is *above* the visible light spectrum in wave *frequency*, another way of measuring light, which is why it is called *ultra*violet.) These light rays come from the sun; some of them reach the earth and our eyes. They are responsible for sunburn, skin cancer and snow blindness and may contribute to the formation of cataracts. UV light may also contribute to the formation of a yellowish spot on the front of the eye (see *Pinguecula*, page 234). Although this is not a serious condition, an irritated spot can be uncomfortable and is easily inflamed by excessive wind, dust, sun or smoke.

Commercial, "off-the-rack" sunglasses of the type for sale in drugstores and elsewhere offer no UV protection. In fact, these kinds of lenses may actually cause your eyes to absorb *more* UV light than you would without any sunglasses at all. The reason for this is that your pupils will dilate when you wear sunglasses; if the sunglasses then offer no UV light filter, more UV light will enter the eye than would enter it if the pupils were exposed directly to the light and were therefore constricted!

Glass lenses block about 98 percent of UV light, and CR-39® plastic lenses can be treated so that they offer good UV light protection. The new polycarbonate lenses offer 100 percent protection against UV light.

Rating Sunglasses

UV light has a wavelength between 286 and 400 nanometers (nm). It can be further divided into subsections: UVC light has a wavelength below 286 nm (not normally considered a threat because much of it is blocked out by the earth's atmosphere before it reaches us); UVB light is between 286 and 320 nm; and UVA light is between 320 and 400 nm.

The Food and Drug Administration has approved a voluntary labeling system to assist consumers in judging the UV protection offered by sunglasses. The FDA has adopted three categories of lenses:

1. *Cosmetic* ("just-for-looks") lenses are those that block out 70 percent of UVB and 20 percent of UVA light as well as 60 percent of visible light.

2. *General Purpose* lenses are for activities like boating and hiking. They block out 95 percent of UVB light, 60 percent of UVA light and 60 to 92 percent of visible light.

3. *Special Purpose* lenses are for skiing and sunning. They block out 99 percent of UVB and 60 percent of UVA light as well as 97 percent of visible light.

Look for the UV light rating on your next pair of sunglasses. However, keep in mind that even the best UV light protection is no guarantee of good optical quality in a sunglass lens.

Protection from Blue Light

The wavelength of blue light is between 400 and 500 nm and is perceivable by the eye. Blue light is considered less dangerous than ultraviolet light, but recent evidence indicates it may be responsible for damage to the eye's retina. Most UV light is absorbed by the lens of the eye (where it may eventually cause a cataract to develop), while blue light goes through the lens and is absorbed by the retina.

Blue light also causes glare on bright, sunny days, so "blue-blocker" sunglasses have been around for a while. Amber and brown sunglass lenses will block blue light, improving contrast in your vision and reducing glare as well as protecting your retina from long-term exposure to blue light.

Protection from Infrared Light

Infrared (IR) light, with a wavelength of over 700 nm, is not visible to the human eye. Its wavelength is longer than that which we can perceive. (Its wave frequency is less than that which we can perceive, which is why we call it infrared, which means "less than" red.) It passes through the cornea and is mostly absorbed by the lens. This light produces heat and is more intense at high altitudes and around bodies of water. It is also produced by the kind of flame used in glassblowing and welding. So, high-altitude skiers, boaters and some glassblowers and welders are at risk for infrared damage, which can cause cataracts in someone who is repeatedly exposed to it for a number of years. Some high-quality sunglasses will block infrared light.

Polarizing Lenses

Many people who spend time around water know the value of *polarizing* lenses. These lenses "polarize" light, which prevents it from scattering—the cause of glare. Polarizing lenses are made from crystals that are aligned in such a way as to change the orientation of the light rays.

The best polarizing lenses are glass, but some quality plastic polarized lenses are also available. They aren't necessarily more expensive than other sunglasses unless they have to be made in your prescription, in which case they will add to the cost of your lenses. Ask your optician about them.

What Color Lens?

The color of lens that you choose for sunglasses is a matter of personal preference. However, most experts agree that gray, green, brown and amber are the lens colors that work the best to reduce glare.

Gray lenses are neutral, transmitting all colors evenly, so you see colors as they are. Green lenses resemble the color sensitivity of your eyes and allow a maximum amount of useful light to reach your eyes. (The eye is most sensitive to colors in the green part of the spectrum, so it will "tune in" better to those colors.) Brown and amber lenses have the advantage of blocking out blue light.

Photochromic lenses like Corning's Photogray® have been around for about thirty years now and continue to be very popular. These lenses automatically darken to a gray or brown color when the surrounding light gets brighter and lighten as it gets darker. The color change takes about a minute to complete. Photochromic lenses don't get completely dark while you're driving because the windshield of the car will block out some UV light. The photochromic process can only be used on glass lenses, so these glasses are heavier than plastic ones. However, the lenses are of excellent quality, and the color-change process never wears out. Prescription eyeglass wearers like these lenses a lot because they can wear them all the time and don't have to switch glasses when they go out in the sun.

Sunglass Quality

Many people make a sunglass selection based on how well the frames fit and how the glasses look rather than on the quality of the lenses.

Off-the-rack sunglasses are likely to have lenses that are made of a type of plastic called *cellulose acetate.* This plastic is usually stamped out into a lens shape and inserted into a frame. The lenses warp, and they distort the light passing through them, which can cause headaches.

With their low-cost materials and low labor costs, these "fun glasses" can sell for between five and fifteen dollars. This low price has led to the unfortunate notion that sunglasses should be cheap and easily replaced when lost or broken. I often hear people say they want cheap sunglasses because they're "just for the beach" — but the beach is where you need the *most* protection!

Quality sunglasses are a different story. They are made from optically ground plastic (usually CR-39®) or glass. Lenses that are optically ground have true curves and substantial "body" to the lens to maintain its shape, and the optics are clear. Plastic lenses can be tinted any color or bleached of color if you change your mind later and want to use them for regular glasses. Glass lenses can be tinted but not bleached.

Glass lenses are almost always optically ground so they are a good bet for sunglasses. Many of the more popular names in sunglasses are glass. Some examples of good brands are: Ray-Ban®, Vuarnet®, Suncloud®, Serengetti® and Rēvo®. They can be made in one of two ways: The color can be incorporated directly into the lens (Ray-Ban® and Serengetti® do this), or tinted coatings can be applied to the front, back or both surfaces of the lenses (the other brands mentioned do it this way). The only disadvantage of the coating method is that the coatings can be scratched off accidentally. With proper care, however, either type of tinted lens works well.

While the lenses are the most important part of a pair of sunglasses, you also need to pay some attention to the frames.

The frames of drugstore sunglasses usually can't be tightened or properly adjusted. The frames used for good sunglasses are of the same quality as those used for prescription glasses. They can be adjusted to fit properly and will hold their adjustment.

Don't let price be your primary consideration when choosing sunglasses. Evaluate your specific sunglass needs (i.e., the beach, bike riding, driving and so on); choose a store that is convenient so that you can come in for adjustments or repairs periodically (be sure someone there *can* adjust glasses); try on several styles; and check for fair pricing. As with most things, you do get what you pay for in sunglasses.

EYEGLASS FRAME MATERIALS

Most eyeglass frames are either plastic, metal or nylon, although researchers are hard at work coming up with new materials for frames.

Plastic Frames

The traditional plastic frame is made from a material called *zyl* (ZILE). This plastic has the unique property of being easy to bend into a particular shape when heated and holding that shape when cooled. This is critical when trying to adjust frames to fit millions of different faces. The material is also available in a variety of translucent and opaque colors.

The 1960s saw the advent of a new type of material called *Optyl*® (ahp-TEEL). This type of plastic weighs 30 percent less than zyl. It can also take on translucent colors. The only problem with optyl is that it tends to lose its shape when repeatedly exposed to heat (for example, being left in a hot car too often.)

Carbon fiber is made by adding carbon powder to plastic, which gives this material the strength of metal and the weight of plastic. Carbon fiber frames are very durable and hold their shape very well. Colors are numerous but are all opaque (not translucent).

Acetate is an inexpensive plastic that is usually used in cheap sunglass frames. It is highly breakable, difficult to adjust and impossible to color completely.

Plastics are still popular for fashionable frames. Each type has its advantages and can be used to enhance your appearance.

Metal Frames

Although many of the metal colors used in frames are a gold color, it is rare to find real gold in eyeglass frames today. Up until the "gold rush" of the early 1980s, most metal frames were gold-filled. However, when the price of gold got out of reach for most manufacturers, a process called electroplating began to be used. Electroplating can put a gold-colored surface on a less expensive metal. Most of the frames made today are still using this process.

Aluminum offers a high strength-to-weight ratio; it's light in weight, yet strong. It is resistant to corrosion and can be treated to take on a variety of colors. Since it cannot be soldered or welded easily, design possibilities are few, and screws and rivets must be used to attach frame sections.

Beryllium is a metal that was developed by NASA and is strong, lightweight and resilient. Because of its high cost, it is often combined with other metals, such as copper, to make frames.

Stainless steel is actually 67 percent iron and 18 percent chrome. It is very resistant to corrosion, and frames can be made thin because of its "springiness." It does not hold adjustments well or allow for easy soldering repair. It is slightly brittle.

Titanium is a metal that has high tensile strength, ultralight weight, impressive durability even when thin and excellent corrosion resistance. It is easy to adjust. It is, however, difficult to weld or solder and is extremely expensive.

Metal frames have excellent qualities and give that "high-class" look to the wearer. Beware of metals that are too inexpensive; they usually lack durability.

Nylon Frames

Nylon is used mostly in sports and safety glasses, the most popular example being Vuarnet® sunglasses. The frames are unbreakable when new but lose moisture and become brittle with age.

Polyamide is a blend of nylons and features durability, reduced weight, flexibility, scratch resistance, the ability to hold translucent colors and a non-irritating surface. It does, however, lose its adjustment if heated.

Rimless and Nearly Rimless Frames

Back in the 1960s, "granny glasses" were all the rage. These were frames that were barely there—only two temples (the part that goes from the glasses to your ears) and a nosepiece bridge, which were held together with a few screws. Any shape could have been designed, though the small, round ones were the most popular. These frames are harder to come by these days but can still be found. Their main disadvantage is that the lenses require holes drilled in them, and the screws used to attach the frame to the lenses often loosen. Drilling holes in the lenses gives them an opportunity to crack. If you have rimless glasses like these, use caution when handling them, especially putting them on and taking them off, and when cleaning them.

Frames that have an upper portion on the front and just a thin nylon cord around the bottom to support the lens are called "rimlon" frames. The cord is positioned in a groove that is cut into the edge of the lens. They have many advantages: They are light in weight, are not very noticeable while being worn and yet are durable if they are of good quality. Their problems are: The nylon cords do stretch with time, so lenses can pop out (though replacing a cord is easy); the edges of the lenses are exposed and can be chipped; and higher prescriptions look very obvious. Using polycarbonate lenses in these frames reduces the thickness of the lens edge.

CHOOSING A FRAME

Ever hear the saying: "Boys don't make passes at girls who wear glasses"? It's so out-of-date now that you may not ever have heard it. Glasses frames have gotten so much more attractive over the past twenty years that they're considered an enhancement, much like makeup or jewelry. To choose a frame for your glasses, I recommend you go to a reputable optical shop and plan to spend some time there. Look for both quality and style, not just price.

Checking Quality

Finding quality eyewear is like knowing real jewelry from costume jewelry. Unless you know what you're looking for and how to judge it, you may be fooled into paying for something you're not getting. Certainly not all frames are alike.

Fashion designers have created quite a stir in the eyeglass frame world in the past few years. The optical industry is suddenly a part of the fashion scene. Most of the designers have some knowledge of what goes into a product with their name on it. However, some just sell their name and let the frame manufacturer take total control and use the least expensive route to make the frame. It's best to examine a frame carefully and ask the optician to tell you about its durability and other characteristics of interest to you.

The quality of frames is evident in the material used, the workmanship, the attention to detail and the integrity of the hinges and nose pads. Examine a frame as you would a piece of jewelry to see if the quality stands out. You may want to compare a few different frames to get a sense of what represents quality workmanship. Also check any warranty that may come with the frame; good ones are under warranty for at least a year or two. In general, expect to pay about $75 to $100 for a high-quality plastic frame and $125 to $175 or more for a metal frame. Rimless frames (metal on top, no frame underneath) will usually run a bit more. A frame that won't crack, peel, chip, tarnish or corrode is valuable and a pleasure to own.

Checking Style

Styles change in frames as they do in clothes, cars, makeup and just about anything else with which we adorn ourselves. There are basic styles that have been around for years and will be here for years to come. And there are styles that make a statement, albeit for a short period of time. Picking the right frame for your face shape, skin tone, hair color, makeup, clothing and lifestyle takes some expertise. Try to find a trustworthy optician who has experience, knowledge and taste in eyewear. Word-of-mouth referrals may be a good source. If you see someone who has good-looking glasses, find out where he or she got them.

Here are some tips you can use to get you started on choosing the right frame. First, you'll need to determine your face shape. To do this, pull your hair away from your face, look into a mirror, and outline your face on the mirror with lipstick (this is a bit messy, but it works!).

Once you know the shape of your face, clean the the mirror and check the chart on page 124 for frame guidelines. The general rule here is that eyewear shapes should contrast face

Choosing a Frame for Your Face

	OVAL FACE **Description:** An oval face is considered to be a "well-balanced" face. The top half balances the bottom half. **Frame:** An oval face can wear just about anything, as long as the frame is in proportion to the face.
	ROUND FACE **Description:** A round face has a large, curved forehead with a rounded chin. The face looks "full," with very few angles. **Frame:** Angular or geometric frames give better contours to a round face.
	HEART-SHAPED FACE **Description:** The forehead is the widest part of the heart-shaped face. Then the face narrows, and the chin is slightly pointed. **Frame:** Try a frame with straight top lines and rounded sides, such as "aviator" or "butterfly" shapes.
	RECTANGULAR FACE **Description:** The rectangular face is long and narrow with a squarish chin. **Frame:** Frames with a strong top bar and round bottom lines are a good choice.
	TRIANGULAR FACE **Description:** The triangular face has a narrow forehead, but is full around the cheeks and chin. **Frame:** A heart-shaped frame is best. Square frames, aviator frames with a straight top or wire frames that are rimless on the bottom can also work well.
	SQUARE FACE **Description:** The square face has a wide forehead and a wide cheek and chin area. The jaw is angular. **Frame:** Oval or round frames add soft lines to a square face.
	DIAMOND-SHAPED FACE **Description:** The diamond-shaped face has a small forehead, a wide temple area and a small chin area. **Frame:** A butterfly-shaped frame is best. You can also try a square frame.

Chart courtesy of You! Are Something Beautiful, La Habra, CA shapes; for example, round frames look good on square faces. Some additional fashion tips to consider: A long nose or wide-set eyes can be de-emphasized with a thick, darkly colored bridge that rests low on the nose. Close-set eyes look good with a high, thin, lightly colored bridge. Thin frame shapes are also a good choice for close-set eyes. A short face can be lengthened with a highly placed temple (earpiece). A wide face looks thinner with a highly placed temple. Full hairstyles around the face call for a thin, light frame. The opposite is also true: With less hair around the face, go for a bolder style.

Take some time in choosing the right frame for you. Don't give yourself ten minutes to find a frame that you'll be wearing for two years! Remember, people will see the frame on your face before they see your face, so think about the image you may want to project. Consider this: Most people have at least six pairs of shoes but only have one pair of glasses, but how often do other people look at your shoes?

Choosing Frames for Children

Choosing frames for children takes special effort and care. Try to make it fun, not frustrating! Approach the process so your child will wear and enjoy her glasses.

Children's frames need to be durable. The glasses will probably be on and off a dozen times a day and should be able to withstand the wear and tear. Many kids' frames have spring hinges on the temples; when bent outward, they just spring back into the proper position. (These hinges are becoming popular for adults too.) To help keep a frame on a child's face, many frames have "cable temples" that wrap around the ears to keep the glasses on. They're especially good for smaller children.

For infants and toddlers, patience is the key to fitting glasses. Let the baby play with the glasses first so he or she becomes familiar with them and feels like keeping them. Have the baby put them on his face if he can; don't worry if the glasses go on upside down! Make a game out of it: on and off, on and off a few times. Let him enjoy the experience.

Older kids want frames that are "cool," and those are often the same as the ones that adults have. Smaller versions of the more popular adult frames are big sellers for kids. Many are adapted to children's sizes by building up the bridge or nosepiece to fit the smaller face of the child. Brighter colors are used because children's clothes are brighter.

Treat your older child with respect and talk to him about the different features of each frame and whether or not it is a good one for his needs. A good optician should be able to advise you here. He or she should make sure the bridge of the frame fits the child's nose correctly, since children's skin is softer and more sensitive to pressure. The temples should be adjusted properly so there is no excessive pressure behind the ears. Comfort is a function of the weight and tension being distributed as evenly as possible. Expect the frames for a growing child to fit for about a year. Don't buy a frame that is too big and expect that the child will "grow into" it.

When the child comes in to pick up the glasses, have him or her look at them first before trying them on. Let her put them on and look through them; then the optician can advise and make adjustments. (Infants and toddlers will probably need the on-and-off game again.) The optician should also go through all the cleaning and care procedures with the child and give her a glasses case, stressing the importance of keeping the glasses in the case when they are not being worn. Bring the child back in a week or two for an adjustment. She can then relate her experience of wearing the glasses to the optician and be reinforced on how well she is doing.

Prices for kids' frames shouldn't be as high as for yours, but don't skimp on quality to save a few dollars. In general, children's glasses should sell for about eighty to a hundred dollars (1990 prices). The keys to a successful frame for kids is: function, fit and comfort. And don't forget: Children who wear corrective lenses should have their vision checked every year.

TAKING CARE OF YOUR GLASSES

Taking care of your glasses doesn't take much time or effort, but a little can go a long way.

When you first get your glasses, be sure they are adjusted by someone who knows what he or she is doing. There's nothing more annoying than having your glasses hurt behind your ears or slip down your nose while you're reading.

To check the fit of your glasses, hold your head down with them on and shake your head firmly. The glasses shouldn't slip down at all. Sometimes it takes a few days before glasses that are too tight start to hurt. Don't be discouraged if it takes two or three return visits to the optical shop to ensure a proper fit.

Many opticians offer little eyeglass screwdriver kits. These kits are OK, but be careful. The screwdrivers are small and it doesn't take much to strip the head of a tiny screw or "inject" yourself with the tiny screwdriver. The best thing to do is to take your glasses in every three months or so for a tightening and "tune-up." If you take them back to the shop where you got them, there should be no charge for this service.

You should always *wet* your plastic lenses before wiping them. If you don't, the dirt on the lens will scratch its surface. I recommend using a one-to-one mixture of glass cleaner and water. Dry the lenses with a soft cotton cloth, *not* with paper tissues. Lenses with anti-reflective coatings need a special cleaning agent that you can buy at an optical shop where you got the glasses. Soaking your glasses in detergent overnight works well to get the frames clean. Even with good care, your lenses will probably need replacing about every one to two years and new frames about every two years. Take good care of your glasses, and they'll take good care of your vision.

Eye Openers

• In 1987 there were 141.1 million Americans, or 58.2 percent of the population, wearing prescription lenses (glasses or contact lenses).

• Sixty-five million pairs of eyeglass lenses and sixty-two million frames were sold through optical shops in the United States in 1987.

• Eighty-three percent of the prescription eyeglass lenses sold in the United States in 1988 were plastic.

• The average price for a pair of glasses in the United States in 1988 was $140.55.

• Nearly one out of six American children between the ages of three and sixteen wears eyeglasses.

CHAPTER 8

Alternatives
to Glasses

When you stop to think about it, glasses are pretty much a way of life for many people. The next time you're walking down the street, notice how many people are wearing glasses. You may be surprised. Glasses are important to some people simply because they correct faulty eyesight, though to others they are a fashion statement. However, there are a few alternatives that are now available to most people who don't want to wear glasses. These alternatives can be classified into two main areas: contact lenses and procedures to alter the shape of the cornea. Optometric vision therapy, which I'll discuss in the next chapter, is another approach to the correction of vision problems.

THE CONTACT LENS ALTERNATIVE

Contact lenses are optical devices made to fit over the cornea of the eye to change its refractive characteristics and improve vision. Many people ask me how I feel about contact lenses. Well, I feel fine about contacts, but I don't have to wear them. Contact lenses are a highly individual experience; you can talk to some people who love their contacts and others who simply can't wear them no matter what kinds they've tried. About twenty-seven million Americans now wear contact lenses, and more people try them every year.

Modern contact lenses have been around since the 1950s, but they've come a long way since then in the materials used, their comfort and "wearability" and in the kinds of conditions they can correct. In general, today's contacts are much more comfortable than those of the past, but not everyone can wear them. Those who have difficulty with contact lenses are: people with chronically dry eyes because of medical conditions or medications they're taking (antihistamines are a problem); people with allergies that make their eyes itch and swell; and people with extremely sensitive eyes who can't accept the thought of having something resting on their eyes.

If you can get past the idea of putting something on your eyeball, contacts do offer some advantages over glasses. Perhaps the most obvious one is that most people like the way they look without glasses. In fact, you can now go one step further than just removing your glasses with contacts—you can actually change your eye color with tinted contacts. But, appearance is not the only reason to wear contact lenses. If you're very nearsighted, for example, your eyeglass lenses will be concave in shape (see *Minus and Plus Lenses*, page 105). When you're looking straight ahead through the center of the glasses, your prescription will be exactly what you need. But, as you get away from the center and out toward the periphery of the lens, a lot of distortion occurs; the lens is of necessity thicker around the periphery, so it doesn't correct your vision very well when you look through it. Nor do you have any correction beyond the edge of the frame on either side. With contacts, the lens stays right on the cornea and moves when you move your eye, so you're always looking through its optical center, where there is virtually no visual distortion.

Until the 1970s, contact lenses caused a lot of problems for their wearers. The lenses were made of hard, impermeable materials—glass until the late 1930s and a hard plastic until the 1970s. And, until the 1950s, contact lenses covered the entire front of the eye, not just the cornea, as they do now. The eye's cornea needs to take in oxygen and get rid of carbon dioxide gases, and it needs to stay wet. The early contacts didn't permit oxygen and carbon dioxide to permeate the lens, and they caused the cornea to swell.

New materials became available in the 1970s, and lenses began to be made that were gas-permeable and *hydrophilic* (water-loving). Today's lenses, which cover only the cornea of the eye, are available in soft and rigid materials (*see* illustration, page 131). Let's take a look at some of the different kinds of contacts.

Contact Lens

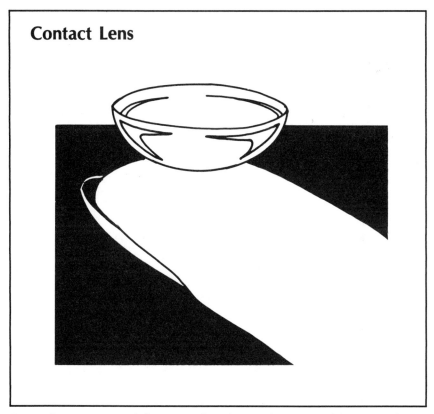

Contact lenses are optical devices made to fit over the cornea of the eye to change its refractive characteristics and improve vision. Today's rigid lenses are usually 9 to 9.5 millimeters in diameter, and today's soft lenses are usually 13.8 to 15 millimeters.

Hard Contacts—the Originals

The earliest contact lenses were developed in Germany in 1927. They were made of glass and covered the entire sclera. In 1937, an early type of plastic was developed for use in contact lenses, but the lenses still covered the whole sclera. These lenses were introduced in the United States in 1938.

In 1940, a plastic called *polymethylmethacrylate—PMMA—* came into use for contacts, which were still made to cover the whole front of the eye. In 1950, the first patent was granted for a lens made of PMMA that covered only the cornea. These plastic lenses were routinely fitted during the 1950s. They were somewhat flexible, but they still earned the name *hard lens.*

The plastic could be molded inexpensively, polished to a smooth optical surface and modified with relative ease (a minor prescription change was an in-office procedure). The lenses maintained good optical transparency that did not fade with time, they didn't crack easily, they didn't sustain bacterial growth (which could cause infection), and they could be tinted slightly to make them easier to see.

These lenses did, however, also have a down side. The material had no ability to transmit oxygen or carbon dioxide, which made it unhealthy for the cornea of the wearer, and it needed solutions on it to help water or tears adhere to the surface. It took some determination to wear these because they were so uncomfortable. However, a certain number of brave souls were able to tolerate the lenses, and they were a definite improvement for those with very high myopia prescriptions. The lenses could sometimes last for as long as ten or fifteen years if they weren't lost (though I don't recommend using them that long).

Today, these lenses are obsolete. The newer materials available have all but displaced them out of optometrists' inventories. If you're still wearing a hard lens material, ask your eye doctor about the newer types of lenses. They're more comfortable and healthier for your eyes.

Soft Contacts for Daily Wear

In the 1960s, a Czechoslovakian chemist named Dr. Otto Wichterle developed a new type of plastic that he thought would be used to make artificial blood vessels and organs until he used a child's erector set to experiment with using it for contact lenses. Called *hydroxyethylmethacrylate (HEMA)*, this material forever changed the world of eye care.

The soft lenses—now referred to as *daily-wear soft lenses*—were introduced to the public in 1971 by the Bausch & Lomb Company of Rochester, New York and marked the beginning of a whole new era in contact lens technology. The material was 38 percent water and was called "hydrophilic" because the lenses absorbed water. They were more permeable to oxygen and carbon dioxide than hard lenses, and the comfort was incredible compared to the hard lens. However, the vision through the lens was not quite as sharp as that with the hard lens, and the early soft lenses could not correct for astigmatism. Also, in addition to absorbing water, these lenses also had an affinity for infection-causing bacteria. The care of the lenses was complicated, often calling for heat units to disinfect the lenses every night. Even so, the incidence of eye infections in soft lens wearers was higher than with the hard lenses. The lenses tended to yellow with age, could tear rather easily and only lasted a year or two despite their substantial price. Still, for those with nearsightedness without astigmatism and the determination to do the disinfecting every night and the lens replacing every year or two, these lenses were wonderful.

In 1976, soft contact lenses became available to people who had astigmatism. The lenses, called *toric* lenses ("torus" is Latin for "bulge"), were now being manufactured using a computerized lathe that could cut different curves onto different areas of the lens in much the same way that glasses are made. These had some limitations also, and large amounts of astigmatism were not correctable, but they worked very well for many people. The first astigmatism lenses were slightly uncomfortable because the lens had a bulge on one side to keep it positioned properly over the cornea. This thickness was noticeable, but the lenses were still more comfortable than hard lenses. They were the same material as the daily-wear soft contacts, so the care was the same, and so were the other problems. Today's astigmatism lenses have thinner edges and are also available in other materials.

Today, soft contacts for daily wear are still popular and can be chemically disinfected (this doesn't usually cause any reaction in the eye) without having to sterilize them with heat.

The average 1989 price for daily-wear soft lenses dispensed by an optometrist was $199. (Ophthalmologists may charge slightly more for all types of contact lenses.)

Rigid Gas-Permeable Contacts for Daily Wear

Patented in 1974 and introduced to the public in 1979, the *rigid gas-permeables* were the next advancement in technology for hard lenses. They looked and acted like a hard lens except that the lens absorbed a small amount of fluid and was able to transmit oxygen and carbon dioxide to and from the eye. This was due to the addition of silicone to the plastic material. This created more lens comfort and better adaptation than the original hard lenses. Because these lenses were not as hard as the originals, they were called "rigid" rather than "hard." Many people who had been able to wear the hard lenses with some discomfort were now able to upgrade to the newer material with almost no change in vision or care regimen. The only drawback to this lens material is that, although the silicone aids in gas transmission, it is not a very wettable surface, so some people experience drying of their eyes toward the end of a day of wearing the lens—more of a discomfort than a danger. These lenses are a good alternative for those patients who can't get good visual correction with soft lenses or don't want the risk of infection that soft lenses pose.

In 1989, optometrists were charging an average of $235 for these daily-wear rigid lenses.

Soft Contacts for Extended Wear

Probably the biggest explosion in the contact lens field was the advent of a contact lens that could actually be worn overnight for days at a time. The only problem seemed to be that the lenses were extremely fragile, although that problem has been significantly improved since the early days.

In 1981, the Food and Drug Administration (FDA) approved *extended-wear soft contacts* designed to be worn for thirty days at a time without cleaning or disinfecting. Unfortunately, this proved to be too long a wearing period and earned the lenses some bad press—not entirely undeserved. In September 1989, the *New England Journal of Medicine* published an article based on a study sponsored by the Contact Lens Institute (a group of contact lens manufacturers). The study noted that the risk of ulcers of the cornea, which can occur with infections of the cornea, was five times greater in extended-wear lens users than in daily-wear lens users, although the rate at which this serious problem occurred was still only 0.2 percent (two out of every thousand) of all extended-wear lens users. All of a sudden everyone was afraid to sleep in contact lenses. Many medical practitioners called for no overnight wear of lenses, but the study did note that the risk of infection increased proportionally with the wearing time.

The members of the Contact Lens Institute now recommend that the wearing time for extended-wear lenses should not exceed seven days and nights for the average patient. They also recommend that some patients should not wear their lenses overnight or should only do so occasionally. People who have a high level of protein in their tears, people with chronically dry eyes, people who have had surgery on their eyelids so that their eyes do not close completely and people who work in exceptionally dirty environments should probably remove, clean and disinfect their lenses every night.

Many patients take out their lenses every night when they're home but leave them in for an occasional weekend or camping trip. This has been called "flexible wear," and it is in fact a term some manufacturers are now using to describe these lenses in order to get away from the controversy associated with the term "extended wear." Today's extended-wear soft lenses are less fragile than their predecessors and can stand up to being handled daily as well as being left in the eye for a few days.

These lenses are more expensive than regular soft lenses— optometrists charged about $256 in 1990 compared to $199 in 1989—but they're certainly more convenient. Consult your eye doctor for advice on whether or not you should be wearing extended-wear soft contacts.

Rigid Gas-Permeable Contacts for Extended Wear

In early 1987, the FDA approved a *rigid gas-permeable contact lens* that could be worn overnight for up to seven days. This material was specifically designed for extended wear and had the optical and handling advantages of hard lenses combined with a wearability closer to that of soft lenses. The key difference was the addition of fluorine to the silicone material during the manufacturing process. This allowed the best combination of gas transmission and moisture maintenance of any lens yet developed. The lenses have been available for some time now, with several manufacturers elaborating on the basic concept, and they are offering the wearer many advantages in lens life and visual clarity. This material allows for a flexible wearing schedule just like what the soft extended-wear lenses offer; it's durable enough to be handled daily, yet apparently safe enough to be left in the eye for a few days. The Contact Lens Institute study on extended-wear problems did not include any rigid gas-permeable lenses. More research needs to be done to determine the safety of this kind of extended-wear lens, but it seems to have great potential for capturing the hearts of millions of contact lens wearers.

The average 1989 price charged by optometrists for these rigid extended-wear lenses was $289.

Disposable Contacts

In 1987 Johnson & Johnson's contact lens subsidiary, Vistakon, released the first "disposable" contact lenses (called

Acuvue®). The lenses were the same as the soft extended-wear lenses, but they were made in an entirely new way that enabled them to be produced and sold so cheaply that they could be discarded after being worn for one or two weeks.

I have my patients wear their disposables for up to two weeks, and I tell them to use a disinfecting solution on the lenses between wearings. (Some patients want to take their lenses out when they sleep, for example, or a lens can come out accidentally.) Some doctors, however, feel that disposable lenses should be worn only once—once the lens is out of the eye, it should be discarded, even if it was only in the eye for an hour. There's some controversy about this, so I recommend that you follow your doctor's instructions, which should be based on the condition of your eyes.

Some practitioners have had some reservations about these lenses and whether or not patients would use them correctly, but the patients I have fitted with them simply love them. There are now three companies making disposable lenses. Call around to find a doctor in your area who works with them, and be sure that complete follow-up care is part of his or her program. Wearers of disposable lenses should visit their optometrists for a vision check every three months as compared with every six to twelve months for wearers of other types of lenses.

The average price charged by optometrists in 1989 for disposable lenses was $398.

Bifocal Contacts

Even back in the days of the first hard contacts, bifocal contacts have been available. But, the original bifocal lenses had all the drawbacks of hard lenses and weren't tolerated very well by a large number of patients.

Nowadays, bifocal contacts are available in rigid gas-permeable materials and in soft materials. The rigid types have a success rate for vision correction of about 70 percent, and people who are already used to this material seem to have little trouble adapting to the bifocal version.

The first soft bifocal contact lenses became available in 1985. The theory of how they should work was well developed, yet in practice these lenses did not perform as well as expected. There have been several different forms of soft bifocal contacts since then, each using a different technique to achieve clarity for near as well as far vision. Unfortunately, none has proven to be the ultimate lens design. Current success rates for vision correction are running at about 40 to 50 percent at best.

But, presbyopes, take heart. Since most of the contact lens wearers are "baby boomers" who are now reaching their early forties, many contact lens manufacturers are putting big money and effort into the research and development of a successful and comfortable bifocal contact lens. New designs are being developed constantly, so it should be only a short time before the next generation of lenses hits the market.

Until the technology creates a bifocal contact lens that will work on a larger percentage of the population, many doctors are using a technique called *monovision* for bifocal patients who want contacts. With this technique, one eye is fitted with a near-vision prescription lens, and the other eye is fitted with a distance-vision prescription lens. If you remember the discussion of amblyopia (see *Amblyopia*, page 69), you know that when the eyes are transmitting two different images to the brain, one of them gets shut off. With the monovision method, when you're looking at something close up, the brain shuts off the image from the distance lens; when you're focused for distance, it shuts off the image from the near lens. You won't develop amblyopia because each eye is being used some of the time. It seems to take about two weeks for the brain to learn this way of seeing, but it works surprisingly well (although not perfectly). If you don't want to wear glasses but need bifocals, you might want to give monovision a try.

Tinted Contacts

For many years, hard and rigid contact lenses have been available with a slight tint, called a "handling tint," that is not really visible on the eye but is just dark enough to enable someone to find the lens if it is accidentally dropped. Manufacturers haven't and probably won't try to change a person's eye color with a hard or rigid lens because these lenses are slightly smaller than soft lenses and don't quite cover the patient's iris. (You'd be walking around with a blue lens ringed by a brown iris, which might be interesting but isn't likely to become popular.)

But, beginning in about 1984, a process of tinting lenses enough to change eye color was developed for soft lenses. The tints caught on and gave lens wearers an additional choice. The first tinted lenses only changed the color of wearers with light blue or green eyes. Then, in 1986, Wesley-Jessen introduced a lens with an opaque tint that would actually turn a brown eye to blue, green or aquamarine. The contact lens industry boomed again. About a third of the new tinted lenses sold had no prescription but were purchased only for cosmetic purposes! The lenses are now available in colors with names like "baby blue," "sapphire" and "misty gray," and many optometrists are offering free trials to see what difference colored contacts can make in your appearance. Theoretically, there's nothing wrong with people wearing contact lenses to change their eye color, but it's important to remember that these lenses are made of the same material as the prescription daily-wear or extended-wear soft lenses and need to be given the same care as any prescription lens. They are still medical devices, not just makeup.

You can now get tinted contacts that act like sunglasses, blocking most visible light and about 90 percent of ultraviolet light. Contacts don't cover the whole cornea, so I don't recommend these routinely as a substitute for a good pair of UV-blocking sunglasses, but water sports enthusiasts find them very useful. Ask your optometrist about them.

Adapting to Contact Lenses

Although the contact lens experience is a very individual one, there are a few common symptoms and signs you should be aware of.

When you first start wearing contact lenses, your eyes go through a period of physiological adaptation; they actually learn to "ignore" the contact lens. (In fact, you could adapt to and ignore an eyelash stuck in your eye if it were present for long enough.) Adaptation to rigid lenses can take up to a week; to soft lenses, up to a day. The contact lens is designed to be on your eye, and most people will adapt to it. By the way, there is no callus built up on the inside of the eyelid when you wear contacts, as some people believe.

You will be put on a wearing schedule when you first get your lenses. Be sure to stick to the wearing times for that day, even if the lenses feel great. Sometimes a problem may exist that you can't feel until the lens is removed. An average wearing schedule for adapting to soft lenses and rigid gas-permeables lets your wear them four hours on the first day, five hours the second day and progressively increases the time until you are up to wearing them all waking hours by the seventh day. Follow your doctor's advice about adapting to your lenses.

Some of the sensations you may notice with rigid gas-permeable lenses include an increased sensitivity to sun and wind, awareness of the lens, frequent blinking, fluctuating tear flow and transient blurry vision. If any of these symptoms persists for over ten days, tell your doctor.

Soft lens adaptation is more subtle. Lens sensation usually disappears within the first thirty to ninety minutes of wearing time. Although these lenses are very comfortable, your vision may occasionally blur and some drying of the lenses and your eyes may occur. Again, let your doctor know what you are experiencing.

Wearing and Caring for Contacts

Rigid and soft contacts require slightly different kinds of care. Your doctor may prefer a particular product or method based on his or her experience and your particular eyes.

For all contacts: Here are some suggestions for wearing and caring for contact lenses.

• Wash your hands with a *non-creamy, non-oily* soap before handling your lenses. Most pump soaps contain creams. Use a clear soap.

• Keep fingernails manicured and short.

• Close the drain when working over a sink!

• Establish a routine of always removing the same lens first to avoid accidentally interchanging your lenses.

• Do not ever insert lenses if your eyes are red or irritated. Wait twenty-four hours, and if those symptoms persist, call your doctor.

• Insert lenses *before* applying makeup but *after* using hair spray.

• Use cream (not powdered) eye shadow and water-soluble makeup. Oils and face creams can cause a film buildup on the lenses.

• Do not wear lenses when using eye medications or when you have an eye infection. Do not use eye-whitening eye drops.

• Check lenses often for nicks or other damage. They may still be worn if they're comfortable, but be especially careful in your handling of them. Order a replacement as soon as possible.

• Clean your lenses, rinse them thoroughly, disinfect them as directed, and change cleaning and storing solutions daily. How well you do this has a profound effect on how long your lenses will last.

• Do not sleep with lenses in place unless this practice is approved by your doctor.

• Do not rub your eyes intensely while lenses are on.

• Avoid any environment that would cause dry eyes, such smoke, wind, dust and so on.

• Remove the lens immediately if a foreign body lodges in your eye. Rinse your eye and the lens thoroughly before reinserting. Do not wear the lens if discomfort continues.

• Do not swim with lenses on unless goggles are worn. Wait at least one hour to reinsert lenses after swimming in chlorinated water.

• Call your doctor if you have a question about the wearing of lenses while using systemic medications.

• Wear sunglasses to help reduce light sensitivity caused by your lenses.

• Do not ever use saliva to wet your contact lenses. Saliva is full of bacteria; it is *not* the same as tears, which are free of bacteria unless you have an eye infection. You can cause a very serious infection by inserting a saliva-coated lens into your eye. You can use water (clean tap water, bottled or distilled water) to wet a rigid lens but only a wetting solution to wet a soft lens. (It's better to put a rigid gas-permeable lens on dry rather than wet it with saliva. Soft lens wearers should always have some wetting solution handy to use in an emergency.)

• Use the cleaning and storing solutions that your doctor recommends. There are hundreds of different solutions on the market today, so be careful if you're considering switching from one brand to another. *Do not switch solutions without your doctor's approval.*

• Clean your lens case periodically by boiling a pot of water, removing it from the heat and soaking your empty case in it for at least twenty minutes. A dirty case contaminates a clean lens.

• Keep a backup pair of glasses on hand, even if you wear your lenses all the time. There may be a time when you are unable to wear your contacts, either because of an infection or a lost lens.

• Get a checkup to evaluate lens performance, visual acuity and ocular health at least once a year.

For soft contacts: Soft contacts need special care.

• Handle the lenses minimally and with the fingertips only. Never handle with your fingernails. Do not crease your lenses.

• Check lenses to make sure they are not inside out before inserting them. If a lens is inside out, it may come out of your eye when you blink, cause irritation or discomfort or blur your vision.

• Ask your doctor about ultrasonic cleaning, which is highly effective in slowing down the buildup on your lenses when performed regularly. (Soft lenses cannot be polished, although rigid gas-permeable lenses can be.)

• Keep your lenses wet when they're not in your eyes. Should a lens dry out, carefully place it in your storing solution or saline for at least four hours. If it is intact, comfortable, and your vision is clear, it is all right to wear. However, once the lens has dried, it has weakened and may tear more easily.

• Do not use water on your soft lenses. Tap water is not clean enough for soft lenses, and any kind of water (including bottled and distilled water) will be absorbed by the soft lens and may cause distortions in it.

• Use only the disinfecting method prescribed by your doctor. Chemical disinfecting systems (including hydrogen peroxide) cannot be interchanged with heat disinfection. *Do not change methods without your doctor's approval.*

Most vision problems today can be at least partially corrected with contact lenses. Much of the success of contacts, however, still depends on how motivated the wearer is.

Contact Lenses

Lens Characteristics	Hard	Soft	RGP*	Disposable
Visual Acuity	Excellent	Good	Excellent	Good
Resistance to Deposits on Lens	Excellent	Poor	Good	Poor
Comfort during First 1-2 Weeks	Poor	Excellent	Fair	Excellent
Comfort after 1-2 Weeks	Good	Excellent	Good	Excellent
Gas Permeability	Poor	Good	Good to Excellent**	Good
Durability	Excellent	Fair	Good	Poor
Ability to Stay Wet	Excellent	Excellent	Good to Excellent	Good
Ease of Care	Excellent	Fair	Excellent	Excellent
Fit (How Well Fit Can Be Individualized)	Excellent	Fair	Excellent	Fair
Flexibilty in Wearing Time	Poor	Good	Good to Excellent	Fair
Tintability	Good	Excellent	Good	Poor

*RGP = Rigid Gas-Permeable

**Rigid gas-permeables vary in their exact formulation depending on their manufacturer, so it's harder to generalize about their characteristics than those of other types of lenses.

In my practice, I prefer to start a patient with a soft lens because of the comfort factor and then move to a rigid lens if the soft lens is not satisfactory; other optometrists like to start with the rigid gas-permeables first and then go to a soft lens if the rigid ones don't work out. If you've been wearing a hard lens without much discomfort, you should probably go to a rigid gas-permeable rather than a soft lens because visual acuity is somewhat better with the rigid lens, and the care and handling of the lenses will be closer to your old routine.

If you're interested in wearing contacts, ask your eye-care professional for the latest information on lenses that are right for your eye problem.

RESHAPING THE CORNEA— ANOTHER ALTERNATIVE TO GLASSES

An eye can be either nearsighted (myopic) or farsighted (hyperopic) for several different reasons. An eye may be nearsighted because it is too long; because its lens has difficulty relaxing its accommodation to focus for distance; or because the curvature of its cornea is too steep. An eye can be farsighted because it is too short; because its lens has difficulty accommodating to focus at near; or because its cornea is too flat. Astigmatism occurs when light is abnormally refracted through the cornea or other parts of the eye.

For the last several years, researchers and eye-care professionals have tried to find ways to correct myopia, hyperopia and astigmatism by reshaping the cornea to correct its refraction of light. There are now several different methods of changing the shape of the cornea. One method uses contact lenses, and the others are surgical procedures.

Reshaping the Cornea with Contact Lenses

When hard contacts were first being fitted, doctors discovered that slight changes occurred in the shape of the cornea after people began wearing them. The corneas of the lens wearers got flatter. It was noted that a flattening of the cornea caused a reduction in the amount of myopia.

In the early 1970s, a group of optometrists got together and started exchanging ideas about what was happening to the corneas of contact lens wearers. They called the process *orthokeratology*—from the Greek word "orthos," which means "straight," and the Greek "kerato" prefix for words that pertain to the cornea. Straightening the cornea with special contact lenses began to look a lot like straightening teeth with dental braces. More research has since been done, and now there are documented cases of people actually reducing their myopia to the point of not having any at all. This process used to take anywhere from twelve to eighteen months, depending on the degree of myopia, but new lens designs and materials have been developed to allow it to take as little as four to six weeks to achieve the same effect.

The lenses now used for orthokeratology are made of the same material as the rigid gas-permeable lenses used for standard vision correction, but they are constructed with a curvature on the back that works to flatten the cornea. They can be about four times more expensive than the standard rigid gas-permeable lenses because an orthokeratology program requires several visits to your optometrist—about seven or eight visits over the course of four or five months. Then, after the cornea has been flattened, you may have to wear a "retainer" lens to keep it that way.

If this technique sounds interesting to you, contact the International Orthokeratology Society to find someone in your area who specializes in it (*see* the list of *Additional Resources* on page 266).

Reshaping the Cornea with Surgery

Since the 1970s, surgery to reshape the cornea to correct refractive errors—called *refractive surgery*—has become popular and controversial. Many people have jumped at the chance to have what they perceived as a permanent correction for their vision problem and a permanent discarding of glasses or contact lenses—only to regret their decision later.

Unfortunately, all types of refractive surgeries carry some risk and involve some problems. For one thing, none of the refractive surgeries affects the *lens* of the eye, only the cornea. Nearly all of us get presbyopia—hardening of the eye's lens—as we age. So, even if you've had refractive surgery to cure your myopia as a young person, you'll still find yourself needing reading glasses to see up close as you get older.

Another problem is that there's no guarantee that any of these procedures will produce the precise visual correction you need. A substantial number of patients find that the surgery has undercorrected or overcorrected their vision problem, which necessitates a second or even third surgery, or going back to glasses or contact lenses.

Still more serious complications are: possible perforation of the cornea (a rare problem); scarring of the cornea, which may cause glare in the visual field (a common problem); and fluctuations in vision as pressures vary in the eye. The long-term complications of refractive surgeries have not yet been completely assessed. But, a cornea that has been through refractive surgery may be less able to withstand a future injury, infection or further surgery, should any be necessary; it may even have difficulty tolerating a contact lens.

If you're interested in having refractive surgery, ask around for a doctor who is very experienced with it and get an evaluation. Also ask other ophthalmologists who *don't* do these procedures what they think of them and why they don't do them. Here are some of the different methods for surgically reshaping the cornea.

Radial keratotomy: The most frequently performed surgical procedure to correct refractive problems is called *radial keratotomy* (that's "radial" — not "radio" — care-uh-TAHT-um-ee), or *RK*. In this procedure, which is used to treat mild to moderate myopia or astigmatism, the surgeon makes a series of three to sixteen cuts in a spoke formation around the periphery of the cornea through most of its thickness, which allows the cornea to flatten out (*see* illustration, page 146). The central portion of the cornea remains clear and untouched to allow light to pass through unscattered. The technique of radial keratotomy was developed by Soviet physician Svyatoslav Fyodorov in 1971 and then refined by several doctors in the United States. It became available here in the early 1980s. Doctors in the United States have had more experience with radial keratotomy than with the other refractive surgeries.

Keratomileusis: Another way to alter the shape of the cornea is to remove an outer layer of the cornea, freeze it and then reshape it on a computer-controlled lathe to predetermined dimensions to correct vision. The removed layer of the cornea is then thawed and sewn back into the patient's eye, where it acts like a contact lens (*see* illustration, page 147). This procedure is called *keratomileusis* (ker-a-toh-mil-OO-sis), or *KM*. It's used to correct moderate to severe myopia and hyperopia.

Epikeratophakia: Still another method for corneal reshaping is with the use of a donor cornea. In this procedure, which is called *epikeratophakia* (ep-ee-KER-a-toh-FAYK-ee-ah), or *EPI*, the patient's own cornea is left in place. A cornea from a human donor is reshaped to specified dimensions and then placed

Radial Keratotomy (RK)

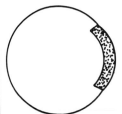 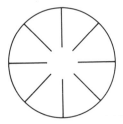 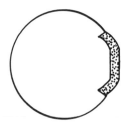

SIDE VIEW
This cornea has a steep curvature, resulting in blurry distance vision for the patient, or myopia.

FRONT VIEW
After the cornea has been numbed with drops, three to sixteen tiny incisions are made in a spoke formation. The center of the cornea is not touched. This procedure causes the cornea to flatten out, which may improve the patient's distance vision. A different pattern of incisions is used to correct astigmatism.

SIDE VIEW
The patient now has a flatter cornea and may be able to see at a distance without glasses or contact lenses.

Radial keratotomy (RK) is the most frequently performed refractive surgery in the United States. It is used to correct myopia and astigmatism. RK can be effective, but it does carry risks, such as damage to the cornea and over- or undercorrection of the refractive error, necessitating further surgery.

directly on top of the patient's own cornea (*see* illustration, page 147). This procedure has been used to correct moderate to severe myopia and hyperopia.

Will eyeglasses become objects of historical interest and curiosity to future generations? Will people look at photographs of us and ask what those queer appliances are in front of our eyes? Although glasses don't seem to pose much of a social handicap anymore (maybe because so many of us wear them), a lot of people are willing to endure discomfort and even risk to get rid of them. Whether you're in the market for simple contact lenses or the latest kind of refractive surgery, be sure you make an informed decision. You only get one pair of eyes.

Keratomileusis (KM)

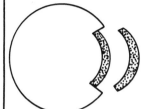 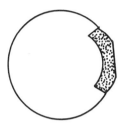

SIDE VIEW
About half the thickness of the patient's cornea is removed by the surgeon. The patient's cornea may be either too steep, causing myopia, or too flat, causing hyperopia.

SIDE VIEW
The removed section of the cornea is frozen and then reshaped on a lathe. In this example, the cornea is being flattened. It could also be made steeper.

SIDE VIEW
The cornea is thawed and then sewn back onto the patient's eye, where it acts like a contact lens to correct vision. In this case, it is correcting myopia by giving the cornea a flatter shape.

Keratomileusis (KM) is a newer procedure than radial keratotomy. It can be used to correct myopia and hyperopia. It carries risks that are similar to those of radial keratotomy; mainly, damage to the cornea and over- or undercorrection of the refractive error.

Epikeratophakia (EPI)

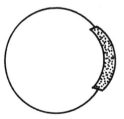 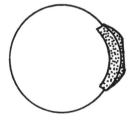

SIDE VIEW
The patient's cornea is not disturbed.

SIDE VIEW
A cornea from a donor is shaped to the proper specifications and placed over the patient's cornea.

SIDE VIEW
The donor cornea provides a new corneal shape—in this case, a flatter shape—to correct the patient's vision.

Epikeratophakia (EPI) is a new surgical procedure used to correct both myopia and hyperopia. Risks of the surgery are similar to those of other refractive surgeries; mainly, damage to the cornea and over- or undercorrection of the refractive error.

Eye Openers

• In 1989, the number of contact lens wearers in the United States was 27.2 million. This figure can be compared with 26 million in 1988, 24.4 million in 1987, 22.7 million in 1986 and 21.6 million in 1985.

• In 1988, soft lenses accounted for 85 percent of the contact lenses sold in the United States; rigid gas-permeables accounted for almost all of the remainder; hard lenses were virtually extinct.

• No need to worry that a contact lens can slip behind your eye. The conjunctiva covers the sclera and then wraps around to cover the inside of the eyelids, forming a barrier to anything that might get behind the eyeball.

• About two hundred thousand people in the United States have undergone refractive surgery.

CHAPTER 9
The Natural Way to Better Vision

Some people want to go to an eye doctor, or any doctor, to get a prescription and be on their way. But, a growing number of people want to play a more active role in their health care and are interested in learning how to take care of themselves.

In this chapter, we'll see how vision therapy, nutritional therapy and acupressure can help maintain or improve vision.

VISION THERAPY

Do your eyes need therapy? If you answer "yes" to several of these questions, vision therapy may be of help to you.

• Do you ever see things blurred at a distance or near, even for a few seconds?

• Do you ever see double?

• Do you lose your place while reading?

• Do your eyes feel tired if you read for an hour?

• Do you get headaches toward the end of the day, especially around your forehead or temples?

• Do your friends see things before you can make them out?

• Does squinting improve your eyesight?

• Does your glasses prescription need to be increased every year or two?

Tomorrow morning, walk into the bathroom immediately after you get up. Take a good look at your eyes in the mirror. Try to describe how they look and then try to describe how your body feels. After your breakfast, shower and whatever else you do before you go to work, take another close look at your eyes. Any difference? How does the rest of your body feel? Again, after work, look at your eyes and see if they had a "hard day at the office" too.

Your eyes do a lot of work in an average day and can get stressed just like any other body part, especially if you do a lot of close work at the office and then come home and read in the evening. Thinking about the questions on page 149 and taking a close look at your eyes from time to time can help you get to know your eyes better, and exercises to relax the eyes and improve vision can help your eyes work better.

Vision therapy is a program of exercises and other activities to reduce stress, guide development of the visual system, improve visual skills and enhance visual performance (see *What Is Vision Therapy?*, page 46). The idea dates back at least as far as the 1920s, although today's vision therapy—it's sometimes called *optometric vision therapy*—is quite different from the programs of the past.

The Bates Method

In the 1920s, a New York ophthalmologist named William H. Bates developed a theory that stress and eyestrain were the primary cause of all vision problems. He reasoned—though not entirely scientifically by today's standards—that reducing stress on the eyes would reduce refractive errors, and he developed a program of relaxation exercises in line with his theory. Bates advised his patients never to stare or look directly at objects, but taught that they should instead learn to "look through" objects. He advised against prolonged fixation of the eyes in one position and advised exercises such as "swinging," which was shifting one's weight from foot to foot while scanning a room, and "sunning," which involved closing the eyes, turning toward the sun and rolling one's head back and forth.

Bates appreciated the connection between mind, brain and eye and said that memory and visual perception were linked. He wasn't entirely wrong—stress certainly *does* influence vision, and there *is* a close connection between the eyes and the brain.

His exercises probably did help people to relax their eyes, but his explorations didn't go far enough and didn't effectively treat most vision problems. Today, optometric vision therapists still use some of Bates's ideas. In fact, the "palming" and "head rolling" exercises in this chapter (page 163) are based on Bates's techniques.

Modern Optometric Vision Therapy

Modern vision therapy as practiced by today's vision therapists (usually optometrists who specialize in vision therapy) began in the 1930s with an American optometrist, A.M. Skeffington, and continues to be refined. Optometric vision therapy combines a series of office visits with exercises for the patient to do at home. When I say "exercise," I'm not referring to building muscle strength, but rather to improving binocular coordination and eye-brain interaction. As you practice the exercises on pages 153 through 163, you won't be strengthening eye muscles (they're already strong enough), but you will be improving the efficiency and smoothness of the muscles that control your eye movements and the focusing of your eye's lens. You'll also be improving the connections between your eyes and your brain and between your two eyes.

Office visits for vision therapy are normally thirty minutes to an hour in length, two to three times a week over a period of several months. In the office, the optometrist uses lenses, prisms and exercises involving light to encourage the eyes to work differently from the way in which they have been working. Some optometrists are also experimenting with stimulating the visual system with different flashes of color to improve vision. The homework sessions involve designated exercises to accomplish vision improvement (but without much equipment).

True optometric vision therapy is more than just exercises such as the ones listed in this chapter; it is an individualized program of progressively arranged conditions of learning for the development of a more efficient and effective visual system. It can be used to improve myopia, hyperopia, presbyopia, visual discomfort, learning difficulties, strabismus, amblyopia, slow reading or poor reading comprehension, poor visual perception, poor sports performance or job-related visual disabilities. But, even in the absence of a complete program, the exercises in this chapter can help improve your visual skills.

These are some of the visual skills that optometric vision therapy seeks to improve.

Tracking: This is the ability to follow a moving object, such as a ball in flight or moving vehicles in traffic, smoothly and accurately with both eyes.

Fixation: This is the ability to quickly and accurately locate and inspect with both eyes a series of stationary objects, one after another, such as moving from word to word while reading.

Accommodation: This is the ability to look quickly from far to near and vice versa without momentary blur, such as looking from the dashboard to cars on the street, or from the chalkboard to a book.

Depth perception: This is the ability to judge relative distances of objects and to see and move accurately in three-dimensional space, such as when parking a car.

Peripheral vision: This is the ability to monitor and interpret what is happening around you while you are attending to a specific task with your central vision and includes the ability to use visual information perceived from a large area.

Binocular coordination: This is the ability to use both eyes together—smoothly, equally, simultaneously and accurately. It includes the ability to *converge* the eyes, which means aiming them toward each other when looking at near objects, and to relax the convergence, which means to move the eyes away from each other as the eyes refocus from near to distant objects.

Hand-eye coordination: This is the ability to use your hands and eyes together in a synchronized manner so that a task like hitting a ball can be performed with efficiency.

Maintaining attention: This is the ability to keep doing any particular skill or activity with ease and without interfering with the performance of other skills.

Near-vision acuity: This is the ability to clearly see, inspect, identify and interpret objects at near distances (within twenty feet of your eyes).

Distance-vision acuity: This is the ability to clearly see, inspect, identify and interpret objects at a distance (more than twenty feet away from your eyes).

Visualization: This is the ability to form mental images in your "mind's eye" and retain them for future recall or for synthesis into new mental images beyond your current or past experiences.

Relaxation: This is the ability to relax the eyes and the visual system; important for preventing and treating eyestrain.

VISION THERAPY EXERCISES

Vision therapy exercises are designed to work on the skills on pages 152 and 153. Here are some exercises you can do at home. It's usually best to do the exercises early in the day, before your eyes are too tired. Don't try to do all the exercises every day. Try all of them over the course of a few days and see which ones are the most difficult for you; then concentrate on those for a period of a few weeks and see what improvements you can make in your vision!

Accommodative Rock

The "accommodative rock" exercise helps improve the eyes' ability to change focus and see clearly at near and at a distance. Accommodation is the process by which the eye changes focus (see *How You Focus Your Eyes*, page 18) and is probably the most important and most often performed function of the eyes. The ability to focus decreases with age, but adequate focusing ability can be maintained for longer periods of time with exercises like this one. To do the "accommodative rock":

1. Put some large letters (such as a large newspaper headline) on a wall and stand back twenty feet (use glasses if necessary to see these letters).

2. Take some small-print letters (such as from a newspaper article) and hold them in one hand. Cover one eye with the other hand (don't close it).

3. Bring the small print as close as you can while still being able to see it clearly. Stop.

4. Look at the large letters on the wall again. Are they clear?

5. Look again at the small print (keep it at the same distance). Clear again? This change in focus (accommodation) should only take a second.

6. Switch back and forth for five minutes until you can clear the distance and near letters easily. Try it with each eye. When this becomes easy, move the small letters one inch closer and repeat the procedure.

7. Do this exercise for five minutes with each eye twice a day—preferably getting both sessions in before evening tiredness sets in. You can also try this exercise in many different situations throughout your day, whenever you find yourself with a near and distant (over twenty feet away) object on which to focus; for example, try switching back and forth between your wristwatch and a wall clock.

Rotations

Rotations increase the eyes' tracking ability and help your ability to pay attention to an activity. Smooth eye movements are basic to good vision. To do this activity, you'll need a marble and a pie tin.

1. Put the marble in the pie tin and tilt the tin so that the marble can roll around the edge of it.

2. Hold the pie tin with the marble about sixteen inches from your eyes and roll the marble around the edge of the tin at a steady pace.

3. Follow the marble with your eyes only, without moving your head.

4. See how well you can concentrate on this exercise for several minutes at a time. Have someone watch your eyes to see how smoothly they are moving.

5. Do this exercise once a day; do it in one direction for five minutes and then in the other direction for five minutes (you'll get dizzy if you keep the marble going in the same direction for more than five minutes).

Alphabet Fixations

"Alphabet fixations" improve your ability to center the eyes on an object in an instant—to fixate on it. This is the type of eye movement used in reading. This exercise also helps with near-vision acuity. To practice alphabet fixations:

1. Cut out two strips of paper. Type or clearly print the alphabet in a vertical column on each strip.

2. Hold the strips about eighteen inches away from you and a bit farther apart than shoulder width.

3. Call out the letters of the alphabet, alternating from one strip to the other ("a" from one strip, then "a" from the other; "b" from one strip, then "b" from the other and so on). Keep your head absolutely still as you do this.

4. Start to spell words by using the letters from alternating strips. For example, spell the word "boy" by taking a "b" from one strip, an "o" from the other strip and a "y" from the first strip. Be sure you see the letters before you call them out! Your speed should increase with practice.

5. Do this exercise once a day for five minutes.

Monocular (One-Eyed) Fixations

Monocular fixation exercises enhance the ability to fixate using one eye at a time. This particular activity is also designed to work on hand-eye coordination. You'll need a string, a small ring (such as one you wear on your finger or a key ring) and a knitting needle or long pencil for this exercise.

1. Attach the ring to the string and hang this apparatus at eye level (from a doorway, for example).

2. Stand about two feet away and cover your left eye.

3. Step forward on your right foot and, using your right hand, try to put the pencil or knitting needle through the ring without touching it. Try this several times.

4. Cover your right eye, step forward on your left foot and, using your left hand, try to put the pencil or needle through the ring.

5. Master this exercise using a stationary ring; then give the ring a push and try going through it in the same manner, only while it's swinging. This is great practice for many sports (see *Visual Skills in Sports*, page 200).

6. Do this exercise for five minutes once a day.

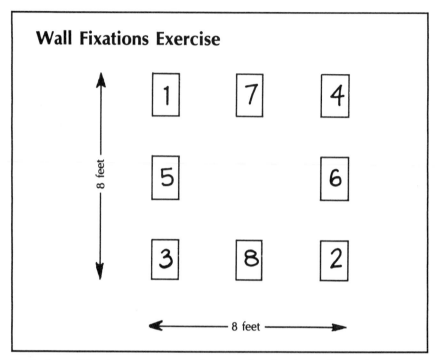

Wall Fixations Exercise

8 feet

8 feet

To do the wall fixations exercise, attach to a wall eight white index cards, each with a number two inches tall in the center. The cards should be arranged in an eight-foot square in the order illustrated. Stand six feet away from the wall in the center of the card pattern. Cover one eye and put a book on your head to remind you to hold your head still. Starting with card number "1," read each card in numerical order, moving only your eyes. Gradually move closer to the wall so that your eye movements become more extreme when you read the cards. Try it with the other eye and then with both eyes together (*see* text on pages 156 and 157 for complete instructions).

Wall Fixations

The wall fixations exercise improves your ability to fixate and your peripheral vision at the same time. You'll need eight white index cards, three inches by five inches each, a felt-tipped marker, a blank wall and maybe some gentle music.

1. Draw one two-inch-high number in the center of each index card, using a felt-tipped marker and a bold stroke, so that you have eight index cards, each with a number from one to eight (*see* illustration above).

2. Fasten the cards to a blank wall in an eight-foot square exactly as shown in the illustration above.

3. Stand about six feet away from the wall and directly in the center of the card pattern. Put a book on your head to keep your head steady, and cover one eye.

4. Starting at the card with the "1," begin shifting only your eyes to each card in numerical order. You may want to have gentle music playing to help keep your eye movements smooth. Keep your head very still and look directy at each number, being aware of the other numbers in your peripheral vision.

5. Move gradually closer to the wall as you improve at this skill. As you do this, your eye movements will have to become more extreme.

6. Switch to the other eye and repeat this procedure.

7. Try this exercise using both eyes together.

8. Do this exercise once a day; do it for two minutes with each eye alone and then two minutes with both eyes.

Marsden Ball

This is a great activity for improving eye tracking and fixation as well as hand-eye coordination and attention maintenance. You'll need a red rubber ball about four inches in diameter, some strong thread or string and a ballpoint pen.

1. Write letters randomly all over the ball with a ballpoint pen.

2. Pierce the ball with the thread or string and suspend the apparatus so that the ball can swing freely.

3. Cover one eye, give the ball a slight push and try to touch one letter at a time as you call it out. Keep your head as still as possible as you do this.

4. Switch to the other eye.

5. Do this exercise once a day; take two minutes for each eye.

Deep Blink

The "deep blink" exercise is designed to improve your ability to accommodate (change your eyes' focus) and your distance acuity. It's also a relaxation technique. If you feel dizzy or faint at any time during this exercise, stop and rest. You'll need a wall and some large letters, such as the ones in large newspaper headlines.

1. Fasten the large letters to the wall.

2. Stand a few feet back from the letters on the wall and, without your glasses or contacts, gradually move back until the letters start to blur. This is the distance at which you'll start working.

3. Sit in a chair in a relaxed posture; take a deep breath and let it out slowly. Repeat this a few times until you feel relaxed.

4. Take a big deep breath and hold it. With your breath held, close your eyes, clench your fists, and tighten the muscles in your whole body—legs, arms, stomach, chest, neck, face, head and eyes. Squeeze these muscles very tightly for about five seconds.

5. Snap open your hands and eyes after about five seconds, exhale quickly through your mouth, and relax your entire body. Breathe slowly and look at the letters, blinking gently as necessary. Stay very relaxed and try to "look through" rather than "look at" the letters. After a second or two the letters should clear. (If you felt dizzy or faint after the clenching-and-relaxing part of this exercise, just do the relaxation part on the next try: Take slow, deep breaths and practice "looking through" the letters on the wall.)

6. Take a step backwards (if the letters remain clear) and repeat this procedure from the new position.

7. Keep going back farther and farther, one step at a time, and see how far back you can go while still keeping the letters clear (no glasses or contacts!). You may be amazed to find that after a few weeks you can stand quite a few feet further back than where you started and still see those letters.

8. Do this exercise once a day.

Brock String Exercise

The Brock string exercise helps develop good depth perception and improves peripheral vision and binocular coordination. You'll need a piece of string four feet in length.

1. Tie a knot in the middle of the string.

2. Attach one end of the string to any object that is at your eye level (you can sit or stand for this activity).

Brock String Exercise

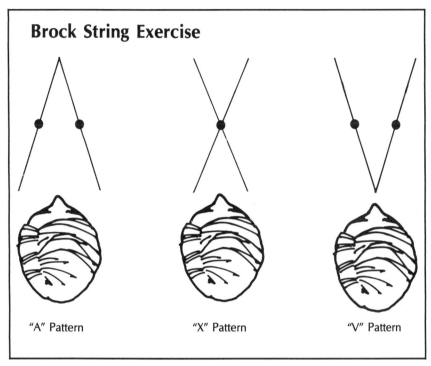

"A" Pattern   "X" Pattern   "V" Pattern

To do the Brock string exercise, tie a knot in the middle of a piece of string that is about four feet long. Attach one end of the string to any object that is at eye level (you can sit or stand to do this). Hold the string between your thumb and forefinger, stretch it taught, and hold it up against your nose. When you look at the far end of the string in this position, you should see an "A" without a crossbar, with the knot in your string appearing as two knots, one on each leg of the "A." When you shift your gaze to the center of the string, you should see an "X" pattern with one knot in the middle of the "X." When you can shift back and forth between the "A" and "X" patterns, move your gaze up the string toward your nose. As you do this, you'll find the center of the "X" moves up toward your nose too, until the string looks more like a "V," with the knot appearing as two knots on both legs of the "V" (*see* text on pages 158, 159 and 160 for complete instructions).

3. Hold the string between your thumb and forefinger, stretch it taut, and hold it up against your nose.

4. Look at the far end of the string. You should see an "A" without the crossbar (*see* illustration above). You should see the knot in the middle of the string as two knots, one on each side of the "A."

5. Look at the knot in the center of the string. It may take a

few seconds, but you should be able to see an "X" pattern with one knot in the middle (*see* illustration, page 159).

6. Shift your gaze back and forth from the "A" to the "X" pattern and back again until it is smooth and requires little effort.

7. Move your gaze up the string toward your nose when you can shift back and forth with the "A" and "X" patterns. As you do this, you'll find the center of the "X" moves up toward your nose too. When you get very close to your nose, the "X" becomes a "V," and the center knot should now appear to be two knots on the two sides of the "V" in your peripheral vision.

8. Practice shifting from "A" to "X" to "V" until you can feel your shift flowing smoothly along the string. As you improve, shorten the string, but keep the knot centered.

9. Do this exercise once a day for five minutes.

Convergence Stimulation

Convergence is the aiming of the eyes toward each other as you look at near objects. This skill is critical for all near-point activities, such as reading. The convergence stimulation exercise helps develop binocular coordination (of which convergence is one aspect) and good depth perception. This exercise also helps your ability to focus your attention. You'll need the illustration on page 161 and a pencil.

1. Focus your eyes (with corrective lenses if necessary) on the illustration on page 161 at your normal reading distance. You should see two sets of concentric circles.

2. Lay the point of your pencil between the two sets of concentric circles and focus on it, staying at your normal reading distance.

3. Move the pencil slowly toward your eyes, leaving the illustration where it is. Keep focusing on the pencil, but be aware of the circles beyond the pencil as you do so.

4. You should begin to see three, rather than two, sets of concentric circles when the pencil is approximately six inches from your eyes. The set in the middle (the one that's not really there) should appear as a three-dimensional figure; the smaller circle should appear to be farther away from you than the larger one,

Convergence Stimulation and Convergence Relaxation Exercises

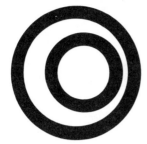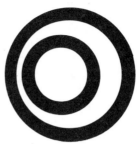

To do the convergence stimulation exercise, focus your eyes on the two sets of concentric circles at your normal reading distance (with corrective lenses if necessary). Then, lay the point of a pencil between the two sets of concentric circles and focus on it, staying at your reading distance. Slowly move the pencil toward your eyes, leaving the illustration where it is. Keep focusing on the pencil, but be aware of the circles beyond the pencil as you do so. When the pencil is about six inches from your eyes, you should begin to see three, rather than two, sets of concentric circles. The set in the middle (the one that's not really there) should appear as a three-dimensional figure that looks something like a cup or a flowerpot; the inner circle should seem farther from you than the outer circle. Your eyes should feel like they're crossing, although they're actually just converging (*see* text on pages 160 and 161 for complete instructions). To do the convergence relaxation exercise, focus your eyes on a blank wall at least ten feet away from you. Then, slowly bring the concentric circles in the illustration into your line of sight at your normal reading distance, keeping your eyes focused on the wall. You should begin to see three sets of concentric circles, just as you did in the convergence stimulation exercise, but this time the circles in the center should appear as upside-down cups or flowerpots; the inner circle should appear closer to you than the outer circle. Your eyes are being pulled away from each other (*see* text on page 162 for complete instructions).

as if it were a cup or flowerpot. Keep the pencil still and keep looking at it. Your eyes should feel like they're crossing (they're actually just pulling in toward each other).

5. Relax your focus after the circles become clear. Look away from the circles for a second. Then try the exercise again.

6. Do this exercise until it is easy to maintain and hold the center image—the middle set of circles with a three-dimensional effect. Then practice it a few times each day, alternating it with the convergence relaxation exercise (*see* next exercise, *Convergence Relaxation*).

Convergence Relaxation

Convergence relaxation is the opposite of convergence stimulation. It's the ability of the eyes to relax (actually to diverge from their converged position) as they focus on distant objects. Excessive near work can cause the eyes to have trouble relaxing, so this is a good exercise to break up your day if you do a lot of reading or computer work. The convergence relaxation exercise helps with binocular coordination (the convergence relaxation aspect of it), depth perception and attention maintenance. You'll need the illustration on page 161 (the same one you used for the convergence stimulation exercise) and a blank wall.

1. Focus your eyes at a blank wall at least ten feet away from you.

2. Bring the illustration of the concentric circles slowly into your line of sight at your normal reading distance, but keep your eyes focused at the wall. (You can hold the illustration just above a point on the wall where your eyes are focused.)

3. You should begin to see three sets of concentric circles, as you did in the convergence stimulation exercise. But, this time, the three-dimensional effect on the center set of circles should have the circles looking like upside-down cups or flowerpots — that is, the smaller circle should appear to be closer to you than the larger circle. (You may see the other sets of circles this way too, in your peripheral vision.)

4. Relax your eyes for a second or two after the circles have become clear. Then try the exercise again.

5. Do this exercise until it becomes easy for you. Then practice it a few minutes each day, alternating it with the convergence stimulation exercise (see *Convergence Stimulation*, page 160).

The convergence stimulation and convergence relaxation exercises should be done together because they are exercising the same set of eye muscles, but pulling them in different directions. If one of these exercises is much easier for you than the other, concentrate on the one that's harder until you can do it as easily as the other one.

Palming

"Palming" is a relaxing measure to use between other exercises and throughout the day. It allows you to relax your mind and your eyes because you're not focusing on anything but blackness. Palming can also increase your visualization skills. This exercise is taken from the Bates method (see *The Bates Method*, page 150).

1. Cover your closed eyes with your hands. Keep the palms over, but not touching, your eyelids. Your fingers should overlap near your hairline and there should be enough room to breathe easily. Rest your elbows on a table. Complete blackness should be all you see. If you see flashes of light, just let them go and allow the blackness to return. You can either continue to focus on the blackness, or you can now start to visualize a relaxing scene of your own choosing.

2. Take a deep breath and feel the muscles around your eyes completely relax.

3. Breathe deeply and slowly eight times and do this exercise at least eight times a day, preferably *before* you start intense near-point visual tasks, such as reading or computer work.

Head Rolling

Head rolling is another relaxation exercise based on the Bates method. It increases blood flow, which increases life-maintaining oxygen, to the brain and eyes—and it feels good.

1. Let your head gently fall forward while seated. Then, slowly roll it around from one shoulder to the the other, making a complete circle. Keep your shoulders level and maintain regular breathing.

2. Change the direction of your head roll. Roll two or three times in each direction.

3. Try this first thing in the morning and again later in the afternoon for a relaxation break.

EAT RIGHT AND SEE BETTER

As you know by now if you've read this far, your eyes are part of a larger system—your whole body. In general, what's good for

Summary of Vision Exercises

Visual Skill	Exercise
Tracking	Rotations Marsden Ball
Fixation	Marsden Ball Alphabet Fixations Wall Fixations Monocular Fixations
Accommodation	Accommodative Rock Deep Blink
Depth Perception	Brock String Convergence Stimulation Convergence Relaxation
Peripheral Vision	Wall Fixations Brock String
Binocular Coordination	Brock String Convergence Stimulation Convergence Relaxation
Hand-Eye Coordination	Monocular Fixations Marsden Ball
Maintaining Attention	Rotations Marsden Ball Convergence Stimulation Convergence Relaxation
Near-Vision Acuity	Accommodative Rock Alphabet Fixations
Distance-Vision Acuity	Accommodative Rock Deep Blink
Visualization	Palming
Relaxation	Palming Head Rolling Deep Blink

the body is good for the eyes, but there are some specifics about nutrition and vision that you may find interesting.

Everybody talks about vitamins these days, but not everyone knows what a *vitamin* really is. The term *vitamin* refers to a substance that the human body needs but cannot manufacture and therefore must take in from the outside world. Vitamins are present in food and, nowadays, in vitamin supplements you can buy at the store.

There may have been a time when a well-rounded diet could provide people with all the vitamins they needed. But, with today's over-processed foods that we further subject to freezing and heating, most of us would be smart to invest in a multivitamin supplement. Look for one that shows it has 100 percent of the "RDA" for each vitamin (stands for "recommended daily allowance").

Some people think that if a little of something is good, a lot must be better. This is rarely true of anything and is certainly not true for vitamins and minerals. Do not exceed the recommended daily allowance for these substances if you take them in pill form; vitamins A, D, E and K are especially dangerous because they are not easily eliminated from the body. You don't have to worry too much about overdosing on vitamins and minerals in food unless you're eating enormous quantities of a food known to be high in a certain nutrient.

If you're under the care of a qualified nutritionist or other health practitioner, high doses—called "therapeutic doses"—of vitamins or minerals may be prescribed for your specific condition. For example, I often prescribe five times the RDA of vitamin A for my patients with dry eyes. But, don't try this on your own. See a nutrition specialist or physician.

Minerals—such as magnesium, copper, zinc, calcium and iron—are also important to the human body, but they are not vitamins. Minerals are inorganic compounds or elements that occur in nature and play a variety of roles in humans and animals. Minerals are essential to the chemical reactions that occur in the body's cells, the balance of fluids in our bodies, to the red blood cells and to our bones and teeth—and they also play a role in the visual process. Some vitamin supplements contain minerals (often iron and calcium).

Last but certainly not least is *protein*. Protein is the foundation of life; without it, no animal or human can live or grow. Protein makes up the fundamental structure of each cell in our bodies, including, of course, the eyes.

Vitamin A

The role of vitamin A in the visual process is essential. When vitamin A is taken into the body, it eventually finds its way to the retina and into the rods and cones of the eye (see *The Eye-Brain Connection*, page 38). Inside a rod cell, the vitamin joins a colorless protein molecule called an *opsin* and forms a compound called *rhodopsin* (roh-DAHP-sin), also known as *visual purple*. When light strikes the retina, it splits the rhodopsin molecule apart—back into vitamin A and opsin. As the vitamin A breaks loose from the opsin molecule, the electrical field of the rod cell changes, and a visual impulse is sent to the optic nerve. In the cones, which are responsible for color vision, vitamin A plays a similar role, combining and splitting off from three different opsins—one for red, one for green and one for blue. The impulses sent from these three kinds of reactions enable us to see combinations of colors.

Vitamin A is also very important in maintaining the moisture in the tissue on the front of your eye. Dry eyes are a very common and potentially serious problem, especially in women over fifty. Recent studies have shown that supplemental vitamin A is effective in restoring the moisture to the tissue. There has been an eye drop developed that contains vitamin A, not just as a lubricant but as a moisture enhancer that assists the tissue in remoisturizing itself. I often recommend it when contact lens wearers mention that they experience dryness in their eyes. These drops are not available at drugstores so you'll have to ask your eye-care professional about them.

Vitamin A is stored in the liver, and taking too much of it can cause problems. Early symptoms of vitamin A "poisoning" include sparse, coarse hair, loss of hair on the eyebrows, dry, rough skin and cracked lips (particularly at the corners). Later, weakness and headaches may occur.

Vitamin A deficiency symptoms include night blindness, burning or scratchy eyes, dry skin or rashes, dandruff and redness around the eyes. Vitamin A is destroyed by liver disease, alcohol, mineral oil, X rays, infections and iron. Because the mineral zinc helps bring vitamin A from the storage areas in the body to the eyes, some practitioners recommend that a zinc supplement be taken with a vitamin A supplement.

Good sources of vitamin A include fish-liver oils and all animal livers, and milk products that include milk fat (such as whole milk, butter, cream and cream cheese).

But, what about Mom telling you to eat your carrots to help you see better? Well, Mom really wasn't wrong on this one. Carrots don't contain vitamin A, but they do contain *carotene*, which the body converts to vitamin A in the liver. Carotene is also present in many green, leafy vegetables and in yellow corn. One more word about carrots: You might think that the best way to get your vitamin A from the carrot is by eating it raw. That may be true for most vegetables but not for carrots. The cells in carrots have very tough walls (that's why they're so hard). Normal chewing does not break down these walls adequately, so although you'll get plenty of roughage, you won't be getting all the other nutrients. Cooked or juiced carrots are the best way to get your daily dose of carotene.

The B Vitamins

The B vitamins are usually referred to as the "B complex," because there are at least a dozen of them (new ones continue to be discovered) that tend to occur in the same food groups and perform similar functions in the body.

Many members of the B complex are important to the eye, but B-1, B-2, B-6, B-12 and B-15 play an especially significant role. These vitamins have their major effect on the nervous system, of which the eye and visual system are a part.

Vitamin B-1, also known as *thiamine* (THY-a-min), is important to the breakdown of *glucose* in the body. Glucose is the form of sugar that your body converts to energy, as it breaks it down, or "metabolizes" it. The retina is second only to the brain in the rate at which it needs to break down glucose to perform its vital functions.

Vitamin B-2, also called *riboflavin* (RY-boh-flay-vin), is another contributor to the metabolism of nutrients in the retina. In addition, it plays a role in maintaining a proper oxygen supply to the cornea.

Vitamin B-6 helps in the regulation of eye pressure. This can be very significant in persons with glaucoma. It also contributes to the metabolism of *amino acids*, the building blocks of protein. The proteins are the basic structural materials of the body's organs and tissue, including the eye.

Vitamin B-12 works at the level of the cell to maintain the the cell's nucleus, the control center of the cell itself.

Vitamin B-15 is a recent discovery, and its function is not entirely understood. It seems to be involved with helping the body's cells make use of oxygen—something the eye's cornea and other parts of the eye must do constantly.

Deficiency of any of the vitamin B complex can cause light sensitivity, burning or watery eyes, chronic eye fatigue, generalized fatigue, redness of the eyes and possibly even cataracts.

Good sources of B vitamins are milk, meat, fish and poultry, eggs and whole or enriched grain products (cereals, breads and flours). Look for the words "enriched" on bread and pasta products; these products have had some of the B vitamins added.

Vitamin C

Vitamin C has been popularized as the "cold" vitamin because of its alleged effects on reducing the number and severity of common colds. But, vitamin C also plays an essential role in the health of the human eye.

Vitamin C levels are higher in the eye than in any other organ in the body. The aqueous humor, which supplies nutrition to the lens of the eye, is very high in this vitamin—twenty times the level found in other body fluids. The lens seems to need large amounts of vitamin C to function, and there is some preliminary evidence that the cloudiness that occurs in a lens when a cataract forms is related to inadequate amounts of it. In a study done at Tufts University from 1984 to 1986, it was found that patients with high levels of vitamin C (along with carotene-like substances) were less likely to develop cataracts. Healthy lenses contain a large amount of vitamin C, while lenses with cataracts contain very little.

The sclera, or white of the eye, also depends on vitamin C to maintain its structure. The vitamin helps to build *collagen* (KOL-a-jen), a fibrous protein found in connective tissue, such as the sclera of the eye. If there is a deficiency here, the structure of the eye can weaken, leading to potential stretching of the tissue with increased pressure from within. This weakening and stretching may lead to an elongated eye and myopia.

Italian physicians have experimented with reducing intraocular pressure in their glaucoma patients with massive doses of vitamin C and have had some success with this method. However, if you have or suspect you have glaucoma, see a qualified eye-care professional before trying any vitamin therapy on your own.

Vitamin C also carries hydrogen and oxygen to the cells. These nutrients help convert food to energy. It is water-soluble, meaning that it gets flushed from the body easily and so needs to be replenished on a regular basis. Vitamin C is destroyed by smoking.

Good sources of vitamin C are oranges, grapefruits, strawberries, broccoli, turnip greens and cauliflower. Vitamin C supplements can be bought in any drugstore or health-food store.

Vitamin D

Vitamin D enables us to use calcium, which is an important ingredient in the bones, teeth and all collagen-containing tissues of the body (such as the sclera of the eye).

It had been known for a long time that people who lived in tropical climates and spent a lot of time in the sun rarely showed signs of vitamin D deficiency (in its most severe form, a bone-deforming disease called "rickets"). But, it wasn't until research early in this century that the true relationship of ultraviolet light to vitamin D was understood. It was found that when the body is exposed to ultraviolet light, a form of cholesterol present in the skin is converted to vitamin D. Of course, the same UV light that gives us natural vitamin D can also cause skin cancer and cataracts — so moderation in everything.

In addition to sitting in the sun, you can now get your vitamin D in fish-liver oils (like the infamous cod-liver oil your mother may remember from her childhood), in vitamin supplements and in milk that has been "fortified" with vitamin D.

Vitamin E

Vitamin E has been called everything from a sex vitamin to a miracle healer, but it may play a vital role in conserving vitamin A and keeping the visual process going. It seems that vitamin E may slow the rate at which vitamin A can be used up in its reaction with the opsin molecule (see *Vitamin A*, page 166).

Good sources of vitamin E are wheat germ, and vegetable oils such as wheat-germ oil, corn oil, soybean oil and cottonseed oil.

Magnesium

Magnesium is a mineral that must be present for many of the chemical reactions in the body's cells to take place. Each cell has about twenty-two thousand chemical interactions that take place thousands of times per minute, and six thousand of these are assisted by magnesium. Magnesium is necessary for the proper functioning of muscles, including the muscles that control the eye. Studies have revealed that the retinas of people with diabetes have reduced levels of magnesium, but researchers have not yet interpreted this finding.

Magnesium can be found in green vegetables, cocoa, nuts, cereal grains, meat, milk and seafood.

Iron

Like magnesium, iron has many functions in the thousands of chemical reactions that go on in the body's cells. But, its unique function is as a constituent of *hemoglobin*, the oxygen-carrying component of red blood cells. Without hemoglobin, none of our cells could get oxygen, and they would die. Oxygen is essential to the functioning of the eye.

Iron can be taken as a supplement and is present in green, leafy vegetables, meat, fish, poultry, eggs, potatoes, dried fruits and in bread and cereal products that have been enriched with iron.

Copper

Copper mobilizes iron for its role in making hemoglobin as well as playing a role in many of the chemical reactions of metabolism in its own right.

Good food sources of copper include shellfish, particularly oysters; organ meats such as the liver, kidney and brains of animals; and plant sources such as nuts, dried legumes, raisins and cocoa. (*Legumes* are beans, peas, lentils and peanuts.)

Zinc

Zinc is responsible for is the mobilization of vitamin A. When there is a lack of vitamin A in a specific area, such as the retina, zinc can help get it there. The retina requires more zinc than any other organ system, and zinc has recently been used as therapy for macular degeneration (see *Macular Degeneration*, page 91). If you have a zinc deficiency, you may notice little white spots on your fingernails.

Seafood (especially oysters), meat, liver, eggs and milk are good sources of zinc. Plant sources include legumes and whole-grain products. Zinc can also be purchased as a supplement, but too much zinc can cause serious cardiovascular and other side effects. Zinc supplements should be taken under the supervision of a health-care professional.

Calcium

The mineral calcium is known as the "builder of bones," but it also builds the supporting structure of the eye, the sclera, and it is crucial in muscle functioning, including that of the eye muscles.

The best sources of calcium are milk and milk products — and calcium supplements.

Protein

Proteins are the building blocks of all the body's tissues, and the eye is certainly no exception. The eye's supporting structures, the lens, the cornea and the muscles are made of protein, and as they break down, or as they grow during childhood, they need protein for repair and maintenance. Myopia is commonly seen in protein-deficient people.

Protein is most easily obtained from animal sources, which are made of protein just as we are. All meats, fish and eggs are high in protein. But, for vegetarians, protein from soybeans and other legumes, such as peanuts, can be used to provide an adequate diet. Tofu is made from soybeans.

Nutritional Therapy for Eye Disorders

Nutritional therapy for eye disorders is still in its infancy, but doctors are starting to take notice of the possibilities. Vitamin C for cataracts, B and C vitamins for glaucoma sufferers and zinc for macular degeneration, along with conventional therapies, are some areas that show promise.

Diabetes, a leading cause of blindness in the United States, can almost be considered a "disease of malnutrition." The fundamental problem in diabetes is the diabetic's inability to utilize glucose for energy, either because of an absolute or a relative lack of the hormone *insulin*, which allows glucose to enter the body's cells in the nondiabetic. The effects of diabetes are far-reaching; one of the more serious is called *diabetic retinopathy* (re-tin-AHP-athee), which means "retinal abnormalities due to diabetes." Hemorrhages and other vascular problems in the retina are the problem (see *Diabetes*, page 225). Nutritional counseling for control of blood sugar (as well as supplemental insulin where indicated) is the cornerstone of diabetic therapy and prevention of blindness in diabetics.

ACUPUNCTURE AND ACUPRESSURE

The basis of traditional Chinese medicine is *acupuncture,* which is a technique for treating certain conditions and for producing anesthesia by passing long, thin needles through the skin to specific points. Although acupuncture has been practiced for about five thousand years, and its textbooks go back about two thousand years, it is only just now becoming accepted in the West.

The technique known as *acupressure* is a modification of acupuncture. Acupressure is a method of achieving relaxation and inducing healthy changes in tissue (such as increased blood flow) by massaging the same points that the Chinese penetrate with needles.

Some of the points used in both acupuncture and acupressure are shown in the illustration on page 173. The points drawn on the faces and hands in this illustration are used by the Chinese acupuncturists to treat conditions like myopia and other refractive errors, excessive tearing, twitching of the eyelids, sinusitis, crossed eyes and other eye conditions. You can use them to give your eyes and head area a healthful, relaxing massage. To give yourself an acupressure massage, refer to the illustration on page 173 as you read these instructions. You should massage each point eight times:

1. Locate a point called *hoku.* To do this, move your thumb up next to your forefinger. Notice the hump that the muscle makes in this position. Press the point that is at the peak of that hump while relaxing the muscles in the hand being massaged. Massage the hoku point on both hands. This point is believed to increase circulation and nerve energy to the head region.

2. Massage with your thumbs and index fingers the two points on either side of the bridge of your nose at the level of your eyes.

3. Place your index fingers and middle fingers together against both sides of your nose near the nostrils with your thumbs on your lower jawbone. Then, remove your middle fingers and massage your cheeks with your index fingers.

4. Use the second knuckle of your index fingers to rub outward following the numbers in the illustration, keeping your other fingers curled under and your thumbs on each side of your forehead.

Acupressure

Hoku

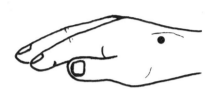

1. First, locate the *hoku* point and massage it on each hand.

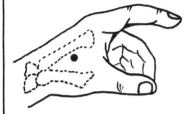

2. Massage the bridge of your nose.

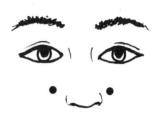

3. Massage your nose near the nostrils.

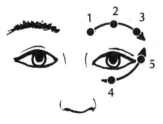

4. Use the second knuckle of your index fingers to massage the numbered points in the order shown.

(*See* text on page 172 for complete instructions.)

Although the future holds much promise of high-tech solutions to vision problems, I believe there will always be a role for exercise, nutrition and relaxation as the cornerstones of eye health and functioning as well as general well-being.

Eye Openers

• The eye contains more vitamin C per unit of weight than any organ in the body. The vitamin C content of the eye makes up about one-third of its weight.

• Between 1984 and 1986, researchers at Tufts University studied about seventy-seven cataract patients and thirty-five people without cataracts. They found that high levels of vitamin C and carotene-like substances reduced the risk of cataracts.

• Many Native Americans of the Southwest used the mesquite plant to treat eye inflammations. The Apaches added water to powdered mesquite leaves and then squeezed the liquid into the eyes through a cloth. Another tribe applied mesquite sap directly to the inflamed eyes.

CHAPTER 10
Eyes on the Job

The information age is here—and with it, the age of eye problems. Human eyes were designed primarily for distance vision—the kind of vision needed for hunting, scanning the horizon for weather and enemies and keeping track of wandering children and animals. Near-point tasks, like making weapons and cooking, didn't take up too much of a person's day throughout most of human history. It's only within the last century or so that vast numbers of people started spending the better part of their days doing paperwork, assembling small parts in factories, reading and doing other intensive near-point tasks. And, it's only within the last decade that millions of people in the developed countries started spending their days staring at computer screens. Eyestrain, headaches and increased myopia are only some of the results.

Even artificial light is a relative newcomer to human eyes. Electric lights have only been around for about a hundred years. Nineteenth-century factories and office buildings generally had huge windows that made use of the sun during daylight hours, and most people worked outside anyway. The first electric lights were pretty similar to sunlight in the wavelengths of light they emitted, although they didn't match the natural spectrum exactly. But, by the 1950s, most offices and factories had switched over to more cost-effective lighting that emits a spectrum quite different from that of sunlight. After millions of years of adaptation to natural light, our eyes suddenly had to cope with an artificial light spectrum for almost all of our waking hours. Research is still being conducted to determine the effects of this change.

Of course, the threat of injury to the eyes is nothing new. Spears, arrows, tree branches and animal tusks probably blinded more than one early human. But, today's workers have to cope with bits of metal and plastic being ejected from machinery at high speeds, toxic chemicals used in manufacturing and the uncertain effects of radiation emitted from computer screens and other equipment. Yes, the workplace can be hazardous to your eyes.

Finally, today's jobs require highly developed visual skills. Your ability to use your eyes efficiently and avoid eyestrain can make your job easier and your success greater. Use the section called *Visual Skills on the Job* that begins on page 189 as a guide to how you can improve your job performance.

NEAR VISION AT WORK

Today's office workers use their near vision nearly all day. Besides taking frequent "eye breaks" and practicing the relaxation techniques in chapter 9 (*see* pages 157 and 163), there are ways to cope with this problem.

Reading

The proper position for reading is at a desk or table that is about waist level when you're sitting at it. Your feet should be flat on the floor or on a footrest. The reading material should be centered in relation to your eyes, not off to one side. Reading distance should be fourteen to sixteen inches from your eyes.

High contrast between your reading light and the surrounding illumination causes significant eyestrain, and I don't recommend high-intensity lamps for this reason. Whether you're using local lighting or overhead illumination, the light should be shaded so that there is no direct glare on your page. If you put a small pocket mirror directly on the page you are reading, you should not be able to see the reflection of the light source. If you do, then you are receiving too much glare. If you're using a floor lamp, keep it about two feet behind the book or paper and about one foot to the side of your work area. A floor lamp for reading should use a 150-watt bulb. A table lamp that is open to the top should be positioned just off to the side about a foot or so and use a 100-watt bulb. If you use a desk lamp, from which all the light is directed downward, keep it at least sixteen inches above the book and use about a 75-watt bulb in it. You can experiment and see what combination of position and lighting causes the least eyestrain for you.

Computer Eye Stress—What Causes It?

While reading-related eye stress was a major concern for professionals and clerical workers in the 1960s and 1970s, computers have opened a Pandora's box of eye problems in the 1980s and 1990s. There are approximately sixty million computer users in the United States today—and at least 75 percent of them have vision problems. The computer is quickly becoming as commonplace and as indispensable as the telephone in the workplace. But, just as with artificial lighting, we may be letting ourselves in for more problems than we bargained for.

A recent study by the National Institute of Occupational Safety and Health found that over 90 percent of those surveyed reported eyestrain and other visual problems associated with the use of computer screens (also called video display terminals or VDTs), and there is evidence that VDT use can accelerate the aging of the eye and perhaps cause a breakdown in the eye's focusing mechanisms. Labor organizations such as the Newspaper Guild and the National Association of Working Women have been lobbying for company-supported eye programs for computer users.

Let's take a look at some of the visual symptoms that are related to work on the computer screen.

Headaches: Headaches frequently accompany prolonged computer-screen work especially if your work station is improperly arranged, your glasses prescription is not right for computer work or the lighting is poor.

Eyestrain: General eyestrain can occur for the same reasons as headaches.

Irritated eyes: The static electric field generated by the VDT monitor acts like a magnet for dust in the air. The result is often irritated eyes. Irritated eyes can also result from visual stress, a contact lens problem or a dry office environment. Offices with computers are usually kept at a low humidity to protect the machines from damage.

Blurred vision: This is most likely due to accommodation difficulties or a lens prescription that wasn't written for computer users.

Difficulty refocusing when looking from copy or screen to distant objects: This occurs when the eye's lens cannot relax and focus for distance after prolonged staring at the near computer screen. It indicates a need for an eye exam and a new glasses prescription—as well as more breaks from the computer.

Double vision: This can occur if the user has binocular coordination difficulties and must use the computer for long periods.

Altered color perception: This can occur after staring at a monochrome (one-color) screen for an entire work day.

The computer causes a great deal of visual stress because it forces people to stay focused at one distance (near or intermediate range depending on how far away the screen is) for prolonged periods of time. The job-related tasks that most computer users perform require fewer eye movements than ordinary reading. Both these factors—single focal distance and limited eye movements—contribute to the eye muscles getting "stuck" in a position from which they cannot easily relax. If you're over forty and your focusing mechanism is not as flexible as it once was, computer stress is generally even more of a problem than it is for younger workers.

What to Do About Computer Stress

If you're experiencing computer stress, there are some things you can do to make your work easier.

Investigate "computer glasses": See your eye-care professional about getting a glasses prescription designed for your computer use. Tell your eye doctor exactly what your symptoms are, how often you use the computer, how far away the computer is from your eyes, what kind of work you do and anything else you can think of that will help you get the right prescription for the job.

If you need bifocals, those of yesteryear just won't work in today's high-tech workplace. Traditional bifocals are designed to have the wearer looking down as he or she reads, which is fine for books and other printed material. However, VDT screens are much higher in our visual field and also tend to be farther away than printed reading material. A bifocal wearer would have to tilt her head backward to position the screen in the reading portion of the lens. One answer to this problem is the progressive lens (see *Trifocals and PAL's*, page 109). These lenses have an intermediate vision range that usually corresponds very well to the distance of the VDT screen. If you only work on a computer for short periods of time, the progressive lens may be a good solution. However, for those who spend the entire work day in front of a screen, the width of the intermediate portion of the lens may feel too narrow. For the full-time VDT user, a single-vision lens that is specifically prescribed for use with the screen at its working distance is the answer. Be sure to give your eye doctor the exact specifications of your work station.

Do the exercises for computer operators: Try some of the exercises listed on page 191 in this chapter (see *Vision Therapy Exercises*, page 153 for instructions on how to do these exercises, which are designed to improve visual skills and decrease fatigue and eyestrain).

Try tinted lenses: If you work on a single-color screen, you can get some glare relief by using a tinted lens to counteract the screen color. When using a screen with green characters, use a purplish red tint in the lens. If the letters are amber, use a light blue tint. For a black-and-white screen, you should try a light gray tint in your glasses.

Keep contact lenses wet: If you wear contact lenses while working on a VDT screen, you may experience a number of problems. First, the air is probably going to be dry, so your lenses will probably feel somewhat dry. In addition to the low humidity, we all tend to blink less often when we read or work on a VDT screen, so the lenses will dry out more easily because of the reduced blinking. Be conscious of the need to blink while using the computer, and keep the lenses wet by using the solution recommended by your eye doctor.

Your contact lenses are designed to correct distance vision, not near or intermediate vision, which is what is required by the computer work. Therefore, your eyes have to accommodate even more than they would if you weren't wearing the lenses in order to stay focused on the screen. This can cause eyestrain and can be very tiring, especially if you have a problem with your binocular coordination. You may want to consider switching to "computer glasses" if you're experiencing problems like this.

Take breaks: Breaks of ten to fifteen minutes at least every two hours are recommended when using a VDT screen. (The National Institute of Safety and Health recommends a fifteen-minute "alternate-task" break after every two hours of VDT work, even when operators are on the computer less than 60 percent of their working time.) I find that many people do better taking a two-minute break every thirty minutes, but you'll have to see what works best for you and your work situation. In any case, be sure to stretch occasionally and look away from your work into a distant space.

Arrange your work station for maximum comfort: If you have any control over your work station, try to follow these suggestions (*see* illustration, page 181).

• Locate your desk to face into an open space beyond the screen so that you can focus for distance from time to time.

• Adjust your chair height so that your thighs can be horizontal. You should be able to adjust the chair for your comfort. It should be well supported with either four legs or five casters. The chair should have a backrest that supports your lower back. A footrest can be used or else the feet should be flat on the floor. Your neck and upper back should be kept straight as you sit at your work station.

• Make your keyboard height about thirty inches from the floor. Your forearms should be parallel with the floor or can be pointed slightly downward if you find that more comfortable. A palm rest can be added to support the wrist.

• Adjust the screen's center so it is five to seven inches below your horizontal line of sight since this is the most comfortable angle. The viewing distance from your eyes should be about eighteen to twenty-six inches, since this distance requires less convergence and focusing of the eyes than a nearer screen. The screen and document holder should, ideally, be at equal distances from the eyes.

• Keep the brightness of the screen about three to four times greater than the room light. Room light should be about *half* the level used in most offices (which were rarely designed with computers in mind). Adjust the screen brightness and contrast to compensate for reflections. Keep away from windows or other bright light sources, including sunlight. Adjust the screen angle to minimize glare. You may even find that avoiding white or

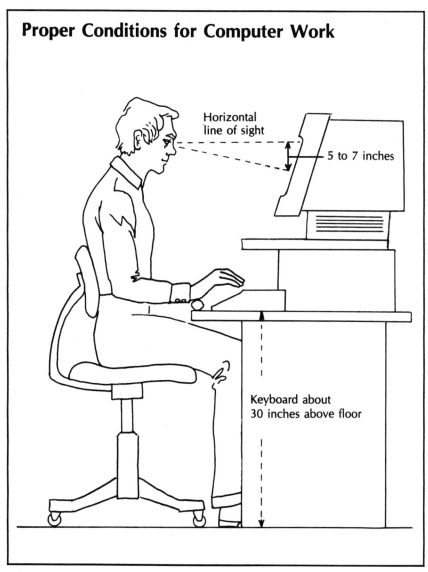

Proper Conditions for Computer Work

Horizontal line of sight

5 to 7 inches

Keyboard about 30 inches above floor

The way in which you arrange your computer work station can make a great deal of difference in how you and your eyes feel while working. Your desk should face into an open area (as it should for any kind of close work) so you can look into the distance from time to time. The computer screen should be about five to seven inches below your horizontal line of sight, and the keyboard should be positioned about thirty inches above the floor. The brightness of the screen should be three to four times greater than the surrounding room lighting, and the room lighting should not be too bright—about half the level used in most offices is best.

light-colored clothing helps reduce reflected glare. If glare continues to be a problem, try using a "glare screen," which fits over the computer screen and is easily obtained at any computer supply store. If you have a private office, try turning off the overhead lights and bringing in a lamp or two from home. This can make the difference between daily headaches and no headaches!

• Consider using a radiation shield. As you've probably heard, computers do emit some electromagnetic radiation, but no one knows for sure just how hazardous this is. Some studies have shown an increased rate of miscarriages in women who were heavy VDT users. No specific eye damage related to radiation has been noted, though it certainly hasn't been ruled out. Since ultraviolet radiation is part of the electromagnetic spectrum, and since excessive UV exposure has been associated with cataracts, it may be found the VDT users will develop more cataracts than other kinds of workers. Several companies now sell special radiation shields for computer screens, although their effectiveness is questionable. You would need a lead shield to block all radiation—and then you wouldn't see anything either! There are screens that block some of the UV radiation, and you can of course get glasses that block UV light (see *Protection from Ultraviolet Light*, page 116).

WORKPLACE LIGHTING

Lighting is something most of us don't pay much attention to—but our eyes are very much affected by it, and our work can be made much easier or harder by varying the kind of illumination in the work area.

General Considerations

If you're setting up your own business or if you're in a position to influence the environment in which you work, here are some tips about lighting that will help you and your employees work better and more safely.

Brightness: The immediate work area—the area on which central vision is focused—should not be very different in brightness from the rest of the room. The brightness of the central field should never be less than that of the surrounding area; in some cases where continuous, intense work is necessary, it can be slightly greater. A lot of contrast between the central and peripheral visual areas is uncomfortable and interferes with vision and work.

Glare: Glare is caused by a light source that is too bright or too close to the eyes or one that is positioned so that it reflects off surfaces in the work area. Older people are usually more sensitive to glare than are younger workers. Bare light bulbs should never be used in a work environment. The brightness and position of lights should be adjusted to avoid glare, and shiny finishes on furniture, walls, ceilings and other surfaces should be avoided. Pay attention to the colors selected for office furnishings and equipment because different colors reflect different amounts of light. For example, black reflects only 1 percent of visible light; dark blue, 8 percent; light blue, 55 percent; and light gray, 75 percent. Consult a lighting designer (they're often affiliated with lighting stores or interior design businesses) to help you pick out the best combinations of light and color for your office or shop.

Differences in illumination: Great differences in illumination between different parts of the work area—such as between storerooms and a customer-service area—can be dangerous if employees must frequently move between these areas. The eyes take only a few minutes to adapt from dim light to bright light, but they take at least thirty minutes to completely adapt to dim light after being in bright light. The danger of errors and accidents is increased during this adaptation period (for instance, while getting something from a dimly lit storage area after being in a brightly lit room). All work areas that are in constant use should have nearly uniform illumination.

Contrasting colors: The more contrast there is between an object and its background, the easier it is to perceive the object. Therefore, contrasting colors can be used to enhance performance and decrease errors and accidents. The moving parts of machines, the edges of steps, hot pipes and so on can be made much more easily visible by having them painted with a color that contrasts sharply with the surrounding color.

Natural and Artificial Light

Let's take a look at the typical day for many urban Americans and see how much natural light we're exposed to. When the alarm goes off for many people during most of the year, it's still dark outside. We hit the bathroom and get a solid dose of artificial light. No natural light yet. We get into our cars and drive to work. If the sun is up yet, some of the light is shielded by the car's windshield. Then, many of us park in an underground garage or deck and ride the elevator to our office. If we're lucky enough to have a window at all at the office, it may not let in very much sunlight. We may get out for a few minutes while walking to and from an artificially lit restaurant for lunch. Then, it's back to the "mines" for the rest of the afternoon. During the winter, it may be dark again by the time we get home. Our exposure to natural light on winter days may be next to nothing.

Does all this matter? There is evidence that it may. Natural light (sunlight) has a spectrum that contains wavelengths of visible light in approximately equal proportions. In other words, the violets, blues, greens, yellows, oranges and reds are approximately equally represented, although there is somewhat more of the greens and blues than there is of the other colors. Of course, the amount of sunlight and the precise spectrum that is visible to us depends on the weather, the time of day and the time of year.

Until the invention of gaslights and electric lights in the nineteenth century, the sun was the only major source of light to which humankind was exposed during the course of a day—and our bodies adapted to it over millions of years of evolution.

Light affects the biochemical reactions and internal rhythms of the human body in countless subtle ways. (Plants and animals need light too, of course.) Everything from the body's sleeping and waking cycles to our hormones, growth, sexual maturation, body temperature, moods and appetite is related to light and darkness.

Deficiencies of light over long periods of time have been known to cause problems for humans. A syndrome of seasonal depression over a long winter in northern climates has been identified and called *seasonal affective disorder*—or *SAD*. It is thought to be caused by a lack of exposure to sunlight.

When hospitals started being built without windows (unthinkable until recent years, when high-tech ventilation systems made this possible), it was found that patients in for a prolonged stay frequently became psychotic from an absence of natural light. Since 1977 in the United States, federal law has required that any hospital room being constructed or remodeled must have a window or skylight.

At this time, it isn't clear just how much *sun*light we need or how close artificial light must be to sunlight in order to meet our biological requirements. We probably need at least some sunlight, or at least an artificial light source that comes very close to sunlight, because our retinas have evolved while responding to natural light. The cones, which are responsible for our daytime vision, are more sensitive to certain wavelengths of light that predominate in sunlight (the green part of the spectrum). Our eyes may even be able to focus on objects and detect motion better when they're in natural light; it seems they're "tuned" to the colors that sunlight enables us to see.

Incandescent Light

The first electric lights were called *incandescent* (in-kan-DES-ent) lights. These lights work by heating a filament with an electrical current until it glows. They are still in use in most homes and many restaurants. Incandescent lights emit a spectrum that is fairly similar to that of sunlight, although it contains more red. Incandescent lights appear "warm" to our eyes and actually *are* warm (they give off heat). Their heat production is one of the reasons they are not used in most workplaces; they make it too expensive to air-condition an office.

People who do a lot of work on a computer screen, or people who must choose and sort colors that will ultimately be used in homes or restaurants, may want to consider incandescent lighting, despite its higher costs. Or, they may want to use an incandescent lamp for part of the day or in one part of the work area.

Fluorescent Light

Fluorescent lights were introduced on a large scale to office buildings in the 1950s. These lights have lamps (the industry's word for what many people call "bulbs") that are hollow tubes filled with mercury vapor. When the mercury vapor is excited by an electrical current, it gives off ultraviolet light, which in turn excites a substance that is coating the inside of the lamp to emit visible light. The exact spectrum of light emitted by a fluorescent lamp depends on what substance or combination of substances is used to coat the inside of the lamp.

These lamps not only use less electricity, making them attractive for businesses, but they are also much cooler, which reduces the cost of cooling a space compared with the cost of doing so if incandescent lighting is used.

Most of us must use fluorescent lighting most of the time because it is so much less expensive than incandescent light. The exact type of fluorescent lamp used should depend on what goes on in the work area.

Different fluorescent lamps for different uses: Most fluorescent lamps emit an uneven spectrum of light—high in the green and yellow part of the spectrum and low in the red wavelengths. Their blues and violets are greater than those found in incandescent light or sunlight, which is why people find fluorescent light "bluish."

However, there are now dozens of different kinds of fluorescent lamps available for different uses, each with a slightly different light spectrum. The General Electric Company, for example, produces about eighteen of them. This effect is achieved by coating the inside of the lamp with different mixtures of substances that produce visible light when excited by UV light. One fluorescent lamp, for example, is heavier in the red spectrum than other fluorescents, and it's recommended for meat markets to enhance the appearance of the meat. There's another that enhances the contrasts among colors by emitting short, discrete wavelengths of light instead of a continuous transition from color to color; it's recommended for clothing stores. Hospital laboratories, where color discrimination is critical, can choose a fluorescent lamp that provides a broad spectrum in each color range, allowing the human eye to make the most subtle color distinctions possible. And, there are others that come close to the spectrum of natural light.

Eyestrain and fluorescent lights: Some people experience eyestrain, headaches or even nausea when they work under fluorescent lights.

If you have this kind of problem, try positioning yourself and your work so that glare is minimized, and eliminate all shiny surfaces from your work area.   You might also try a slight rose tint in your glasses to enhance the red end of the color spectrum that is weak in the fluorescent lights most offices use.

Some people are bothered by fluorescent lights because they perceive a flicker in them. (Others never seem to see this flicker under any circumstances.) When fluorescent lamps are used with alternating current—as they all are in the United States— the lamp receives its electricity in cycles; a peak surge of electrical current is followed by a lull at the rate of sixty cycles per second. When fluorescent lamps get old or when they are improperly maintained, this cyclic electrical current may cause them to flicker at a rate that is perceptible to at least some human eyes.

To minimize the flicker in fluorescent lights, be sure that lamps are properly maintained and are changed before they wear out. You can also arrange the lamps in a two-lamp fixture so that they are cycled opposite each other with respect to the current; in other words, one lamp is being electrically stimulated while the other is in its "off" phase, which decreases the possibility of a flicker being noticed. A lighting specialist or electrical engineer should be able to help you with this kind of problem.

Health, Body Rhythms and Artificial Light

It is clear that people need light at regular hours of the day in order to function properly. What is not clear is whether this light must come only from the sun to meet human biochemical needs. In fact, specialized fluorescent lamps with varying light spectra have been used to treat people with seasonal affective disorder, psoriasis and jaundice, and may soon be used to treat people with jet lag. There may one day be a cost-effective electric light that emits a spectrum identical to sunlight.

However, for now, most of us work under limited-spectrum artificial light that is quite different from natural light. This kind of light probably doesn't meet all our light needs, so we should try to get a dose of natural light at lunchtime and on weekends. Most of us don't need much coaxing to do this.

EYE SAFETY ON THE JOB

So, office workers may be straining their eyes all day, but you're a truck driver or a construction worker or a gardener, so you don't have to worry about your eyes—right? Wrong. Occupational hazards for the eyes exist in almost all occupations; they're just a little different in each one.

Anyone who works in construction, landscaping or manufacturing (as well as other occupations—from zookeepers to dentists and chemists) should be aware of the importance of safety glasses on the job (*see* illustration, page 188). It only takes one small fragment flying in the wrong direction or one splashed chemical to destroy your eyesight. For many years, safety

Safety Glasses for Work

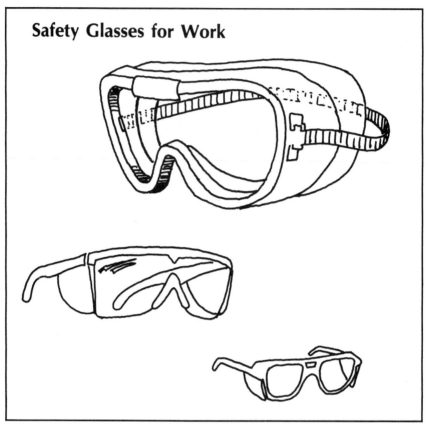

Three styles of safety glasses are shown. Polycarbonate safety lenses give the same protection against flying fragments as the older "industrial-thickness" glass lenses, and they protect against ultraviolet light as well.

glasses were made of "industrial-thickness" glass lenses. Today's polycarbonate safety lenses give the same protection without the thickness—and they also protect against ultraviolet radiation.

Gardeners and anyone who works outdoors should wear glasses with ultraviolet protection as well as protection against flying particles because cataracts and other eye damage can result with excessive exposure to UV light. Drivers of trucks and other vehicles can get some UV protection from the windshield, but they should still wear sunglasses during the peak sun hours of the day and while driving into a sunset.

Glassblowers, welders and people who work at high altitudes or around water need lenses with infrared protection.

Safety First

Many an emergency-room doctor who can't save an eye has heard the phrase "I know I should have, but I was in a hurry." Don't become a statistic.

Wear the safety glasses, goggles or shield provided for you. If you don't have this equipment, make sure you get it.

Never remove safety guards from machinery just to make your work easier or faster. Think how much more difficult your job would be with one eye.

Know the location of first-aid equipment and emergency medical services in your work area. Most high-risk areas, such as chemistry labs, have special equipment for washing chemicals out of the eye. Most such areas also have standard procedures to follow to get help in an emergency. Find out what they are.

Wear lenses that protect against ultraviolet radiation if you work outdoors or with computers. You can get glasses or contact lenses that do this. Some evidence suggests you should also protect yourself from ultraviolet radiation if you're a regular computer user.

Wear lenses that protect against infrared radiation if you work in certain occupations. People who work around welding or glassblowing equipment, and people who work at high altitudes or around water, should have infrared-protecting lenses.

VISUAL SKILLS ON THE JOB

Almost all occupations require visual skills. Without them, many jobs would be extremely difficult, if not impossible, to do.

You can help yourself with the exercises listed in the following pages. You'll find the instructions for them in chapter 9, beginning on page 153. For a more complete diagnosis and individualized vision therapy program, consult an optometrist who specializes in vision therapy.

Exercises for Your Job

Occupation	Visual Skills Needed	Exercises
Executive, Professional	Near-Vision Acuity	Accommodative Rock Alphabet Fixations
	Accommodation	Accommodative Rock Deep Blink
	Fixation	Marsden Ball Alphabet Fixations Wall Fixations Monocular Fixations
	Binocular Coordination	Brock String Convergence Stimulation Convergence Relaxation
	Maintaining Attention	Rotations Marsden Ball Convergence Stimulation Convergence Relaxation
	Visualization	Palming
	Relaxation	Palming Head Rolling Deep Blink
Secretary	Near-Vision Acuity	Accommodative Rock Alphabet Fixations
	Accommodation	Accommodative Rock Deep Blink
	Fixation	Marsden Ball Alphabet Fixations Wall Fixations Monocular Fixations
	Binocular Coordination	Brock String Convergence Stimulation Convergence Relaxation
	Hand-Eye Coordination	Monocular Fixations Marsden Ball
	Maintaining Attention	Rotations Marsden Ball Convergence Stimulation Convergence Relaxation
	Relaxation	Palming Head Rolling Deep Blink

Computer Operator	Fixation	Marsden Ball Alphabet Fixations Wall Fixations Monocular Fixations
	Binocular Coordination	Brock String Convergence Stimulation Convergence Relaxation
	Maintaining Attention	Rotations Marsden Ball Convergence Stimulation Convergence Relaxation
	Accommodation	Accommodative Rock Deep Blink
	Near-Vision Acuity	Accommodative Rock Alphabet Fixations
	Relaxation	Palming Head Rolling Deep Blink
Truck Driver	Tracking	Rotations Marsden Ball
	Fixation	Marsden Ball Alphabet Fixations Wall Fixations Monocular Fixations
	Accommodation	Accommodative Rock Deep Blink
	Depth Perception	Brock String Convergence Stimulation Convergence Relaxation
	Peripheral Vision	Wall Fixations Brock String
	Binocular Coordination	Brock String Convergence Stimulation Convergence Relaxation
	Maintaining Attention	Rotations Marsden Ball Convergence Stimulation Convergence Relaxation
	Distance-Vision Acuity	Accommodative Rock Deep Blink

Construction Worker	Fixation	Marsden Ball Alphabet Fixations Wall Fixations Monocular Fixations
	Accommodation	Accommodative Rock Deep Blink
	Depth Perception	Brock String Convergence Stimulation Convergence Relaxation
	Binocular Coordination	Brock String Convergence Stimulation Convergence Relaxation
	Hand-Eye Coordination	Monocular Fixations Marsden Ball
	Maintaining Attention	Rotations Marsden Ball Convergence Stimulation Convergence Relaxation
	Near-Vision Acuity	Accommodative Rock Alphabet Fixations
	Visualization	Palming
Assembly-Line Worker	Tracking	Rotations Marsden Ball
	Fixation	Marsden Ball Alphabet Fixations Wall Fixations Monocular Fixations
	Accommodation	Accommodative Rock Deep Blink
	Depth Perception	Brock String Convergence Stimulation Convergence Relaxation
	Binocular Coordination	Brock String Convergence Stimulation Convergence Relaxation
	Hand-Eye Coordination	Monocular Fixations Marsden Ball
	Maintaining Attention	Rotations Marsden Ball Convergence Stimulation Convergence Relaxation
	Near-Vision Acuity	Accommodative Rock Alphabet Fixations

	Relaxation	Palming Head Rolling Deep Blink
Waiter, Waitress	Fixation	Marsden Ball Alphabet Fixations Wall Fixations Monocular Fixations
	Accommodation	Accommodative Rock Deep Blink
	Depth Perception	Brock String Convergence Stimulation Convergence Relaxation
	Peripheral Vision	Wall Fixations Brock String
	Binocular Coordination	Brock String Convergence Stimulation Convergence Relaxation
	Hand-Eye Coordination	Monocular Fixations Marsden Ball
	Near-Vision Acuity	Accommodative Rock Alphabet Fixations
Firefighter	Tracking	Rotations Marsden Ball
	Fixation	Marsden Ball Alphabet Fixations Wall Fixations Monocular Fixations
	Depth Perception	Brock String Convergence Stimulation Convergence Relaxation
	Peripheral Vision	Wall Fixations Brock String
	Binocular Coordination	Brock String Convergence Stimulation Convergence Relaxation
	Hand-Eye Coordination	Monocular Fixations Marsden Ball
	Distance-Vision Acuity	Accommodative Rock Deep Blink
Police Officer	Tracking	Rotations Marsden Ball

	Fixation	Marsden Ball
		Alphabet Fixations
		Wall Fixations
		Monocular Fixations
	Accommodation	Accommodative Rock
		Deep Blik
	Depth Perception	Brock String
		Convergence Stimulation
		Convergence Relaxation
	Peripheral Vision	Wall Fixations
		Brock String
	Hand-Eye Coordination	Monocular Fixations
		Marsden Ball
	Distance-Vision Acuity	Accommodative Rock
		Deep Blink
Pilot	Tracking	Rotations
		Marsden Ball
	Fixation	Marsden Ball
		Alphabet Fixations
		Wall Fixations
		Monocular Fixations
	Accommodation	Accommodative Rock
		Deep Blink
	Depth Perception	Brock String
		Convergence Stimulation
		Convergence Relaxation
	Peripheral Vision	Wall Fixations
		Brock String
	Binocular Coordination	Brock String
		Convergence Stimulation
		Convergence Relaxation
	Hand-Eye Coordination	Monocular Fixations
		Marsden Ball
	Maintaining Attention	Rotations
		Marsden Ball
		Convergence Stimulation
		Convergence Relaxation
	Near-Vision Acuity	Accommodative Rock
		Alphabet Fixations
	Distance-Vision Acuity	Accommodative Rock
		Deep Blink
	Visualization	Palming

Computers, chemicals, flying fragments, artificial lighting and even excessive sunlight can cause problems for working eyes. Protecting your eyes from injury and strain and improving your visual skills are smart career moves.

Eye Openers

• You won't injure your eyes by reading in poor light, but you will strain them, which may cause a headache. This best cure for this type of eyestrain is to rest your eyes periodically by focusing into the distance—and improve the lighting in your office.

• Those who burn the midnight oil should know that reading in bed is not good for your eyes. It's almost impossible to get into a good position for visual input while lying in bed. And, we usually read in bed when our eyes are the most tired.

• Incandescent lighting requires about three times the amount of electrical energy and produces about three times the amount of heat that fluorescent lighting does.

• The National Safety Council reports that approximately 5 percent of injuries resulting from work-related accidents are injuries to the eyes. There are about one hundred thousand such injuries each year in the United States.

• There is no truth to the rumor that electrical sparks or sparks from welding equipment cause contact lenses to become fused to workers' eyes.

CHAPTER 11

Eyes in Sports

One reason I believe we can work so well as a nation is that we play so well. A unique aspect of American life that sets us apart from many other countries is our dedication to sports. One look at the number of American medal winners from any year of Olympic Games will show how dedicated Americans are to superior sports achievement.

Of course, sports are an area where eye safety is of the utmost importance. Flying objects (usually balls) and water, sun and wind can all damage the eyes of sports enthusiasts. Fortunately, most eye accidents can be prevented with the right care and equipment.

You might think that physical conditioning is the only key to successful achievement in sports, but without our eyes to guide us, sports performance would suffer greatly. Good visual skills are essential in almost all sports. Baseball, basketball, football, tennis and all the other American favorites require well-honed visual skills that you can improve with some vision therapy exercises (see *Visual Skills in Sports*, page 200). I sometimes think that one of the reasons golf is so popular with older people is that, although it requires certain kinds of visual skills, it doesn't require much visual accommodation, which is difficult for us as we age.

CAUTION—FLYING OBJECTS, WATER, SUN AND WIND

All sports require attention to eye safety, although the problems are a little different in each sport. Taking just a few precautions can save you a lifetime of suffering from an unnecessary eye injury.

Protective Eyewear for Sports

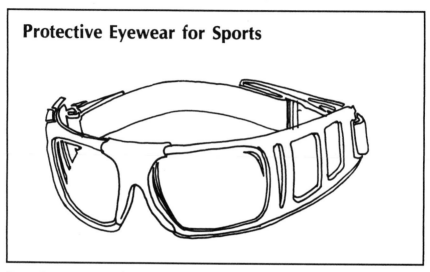

Protective eyewear such as these goggles can save your eyes from injury by flying balls, rackets and bats. High-risk contact or impact sports, such as hockey, football and some positions in baseball (such as catcher and umpire) require a helmet and face mask for maximum protection.

Flying Objects

Football, baseball and racket sports present obvious risks to the eyes in the form of flying balls—and an occasional flying racket or other object. (Someone once asked me how he should protect his eyes while boxing. I told him the only sure way to do this was to stay out of his opponent's reach.) Protective eyewear is a must for these sports (*see* illustration above).

Federal standards for protective eyewear have been developed by the American National Standard Institute (ANSI). These standards require a material to withstand certain kinds of impact and abuse under performance conditions. Each particular sport or use has a particular standard by which it is tested. When purchasing protective eyewear, ask whether it has met the ANSI standards. If it does, the eyewear should have a "Z87" marked on it (referring to the standard known as ANSI Z87.1-1989).

The ANSI considers sports that are "low-risk" to be those in which there is a minimal chance of contact or impact between players, such as track and field, swimming and gymnastics. Moderate—to high-risk sports are those where contact between players and between ball and player occur, such as racket sports, hockey, lacrosse, soccer, baseball, basketball, football and volleyball. Extreme-risk sports are the "combative" sports, such as karate and boxing.

The following guidelines will help you to select appropriate eye protection for various sports and recreational activities.

Normal ("street-wear") frames with two-millimeter polycarbonate lenses: These are acceptable protection for daily use by active people and are satisfactory for athletes who need vision correction while they participate in low-risk sports (such as track and field, swimming and gymnastics).

Sports frames with three-millimeter polycarbonate lenses: These are recommended for people who need vision correction during moderate—to high-risk sports that do not involve direct contact between the players (for example, racket sports, basketball and baseball). For athletes who need vision correction during high-risk contact sports, these should be worn in combination with a face mask or helmet.

Molded polycarbonate frames and lenses (nonprescription): These are suggested for contact lens wearers or athletes who do not need vision correction who participate in moderate to high-risk, non-contact sports (such as racket sports, basetball and baseball). They can be used in combination with a face mask or helmet for additional protection in high-risk contact sports.

Face masks and helmets: These are required for use in high-risk contact or impact sports (such as hockey, football and some positions in baseball, such as catcher or umpire).

Water, Sun and Wind

Water sports—swimming, diving, surfing and sailing—pose their own hazards to the eyes in the form of irritation from chlorine or salt water, ultraviolet and infrared light and glare.

People who need vision correction often ask my advice about swimming. It's pretty hard to swim with glasses on, but you can get prescription goggles that work very well.

A lot of people ask me about wearing contact lenses while swimming. Although contact lens manufacturers recommend against swimming with contacts in, it may be safe to disregard this advice *if* you take appropriate precautions. If you wear gas-permeable lenses, the main problem is that they're prone to floating away. However, soft contacts absorb water, including the water you're swimming in—which may be full of bacteria, salt or chlorine. Swimming in a fresh-water pond will allow a lot of bacteria to enter the lens, so it's important that you remove the lens right after swimming and disinfect it properly. If you're swimming or surfing in salty ocean water, use lubricating drops before and after swimming to neutralize the effects of the high salt concentration. Remove and disinfect the lens as soon as possible afterwards. Swimming in chlorinated pools will usually cause the lenses to sting your eyes, so lubricating with drops or saline solution is recommended immediately after swimming. Then, remove the lenses and disinfect them within thirty minutes as a precaution against infection.

Swimming with goggles over your contact lenses will allow you to use your lenses safely and reduce the amount of water coming into contact with your lenses. If you prefer not to use your contact lenses while swimming, prescription goggles are available at many optical stores and are a good alternative to your contacts.

Sun and wind are two other problems athletes face, on the water and elsewhere. You can actually burn your retinas or corneas and sustain serious, permanent eye damage from staring at the sun on reflected water (while sailing or surfing, for example). A good pair of UV-blocking sunglasses or goggles or at least UV-blocking contact lenses will reduce a lot of the risk of this kind of problem.

The danger of infrared radiation is mostly the heat generated by it; burns can occur without your realizing what is happening. Most high-quality sunglasses will help reduce the infrared as well as the ultraviolet radiation, but if you spend a significant amount of time near bodies of water or in high altitudes in the snow you may want to invest in special sunglasses that filter out infrared radiation. Bolle® and Rēvo® are two available brands.

Wind can be a problem to athletes because of the drying effect on the eyes, especially if contact lenses are worn. Wind can dry out contact lenses or even blow them out of the eye. Also, debris can be more easily trapped behind a lens in windy conditions. Wear glasses or goggles with wraparound lenses on windy days, and be sure to use and carry plenty of wetting solution if you have contacts.

VISUAL SKILLS IN SPORTS

Without good vision, good athletic performance is impossible. Consider our national pastime—baseball. The ability to spot that small white ball from about three hundred feet takes superb visual acuity. Accurate depth perception and binocular coordination enable a player to hit and catch that ball. Can you imagine trying to hit a ball without knowing how far away from you it is? If you watch baseball outfielders, you may notice that the good ones start running for the ball "at the crack of the bat." Their visual acuity and depth perception let them judge whether the ball is going over their heads or in front of them. Their well-developed peripheral vision tells them where they are in relation to the other players without their having to look directly at them. Hand-eye coordination is crucial to all sports, and it is certainly the critical factor in batting. The eyes receive the image of the ball as it comes toward the batter; the optic nerve sends the information to the visual cortex at the back of the brain; then it goes the motor cortex, which tells the muscles of the arm what to do to hit the ball. And, all this happens in about one-fiftieth of a second!

And, what about basketball? Throwing a ball through a hoop from varying distances and angles requires excellent depth perception. Knowing how to dribble the ball and, at the same time to break through players who are trying to stop you, takes good hand-eye coordination and peripheral vision. Recently, I saw an exhibition basketball game where they wanted to handicap the winning team. To do so, they made the team wear trick glasses that partially obscured their vision. Needless to say, passes weren't received, balls were fumbled, and no baskets were made while the glasses were on—and the other team won.

What can you do to improve your vision for your favorite sport? Try the exercises listed in the section that begins below; the instructions for the exercises are in chapter 9, beginning on page 153. These are techniques you can easily do at home. To further enhance your athletic performance through enhancing your visual skills, see an optometrist who specializes in vision therapy or sports vision so that an individualized program can be designed for you.

Exercises for Your Sport

Sport	Visual Skills Needed	Exercises
Baseball	Tracking	Rotations Marsden Ball
	Hand-Eye Coordination	Monocular Fixations Marsden Ball

	Accommodative Rock	Accommodative Rock Deep Blink
	Depth Perception	Brock String Convergence Stimulation Convergence Relaxation
	Peripheral Vision	Wall Fixations Brock String
	Binocular Coordination	Brock String Convergence Stimulation Convergence Relaxation
	Distance-Vision Acuity	Accommodative Rock Deep Blink
	Visualization	Palming
	Relaxation	Palming Head Rolling Deep Blink
Football	Tracking	Rotations Marsden Ball
	Accommodation	Accommodative Rock Deep Blink
	Depth Perception	Brock String Convergence Stimulation Convergence Relaxation
	Hand-Eye Coordination	Monocular Fixations Marsden Ball
	Peripheral Vision	Wall Fixations Brock String
	Binocular Coordination	Brock String Convergence Stimulation Convergence Relaxation
	Maintaining Attention	Rotations Marsden Ball Convergence Stimulation Convergence Relaxation
	Near-Vision Acuity	Accommodative Rock Alphabet Fixations
	Distance-Vision Acuity	Accommodative Rock Deep Blink
	Visualization	Palming
Basketball	Tracking	Rotations Marsden Ball

	Fixation	Marsden Ball Alphabet Fixations Wall Fixations Monocular Fixations
	Accommodation	Accommodative Rock Deep Blink
	Depth Perception	Brock String Convergence Stimulation Convergence Relaxation
	Hand-Eye Coordination	Monocular Fixations Marsden Ball
	Peripheral Vision	Wall Fixations Brock String
	Binocular Coordination	Brock String Convergence Stimulation Convergence Relaxation
	Maintaining Attention	Rotations Marsden Ball Convergence Stimulation Convergence Relaxation
	Distance-Vision Acuity	Accommodative Rock Deep Blink
	Visualization	Palming
Soccer	Tracking	Rotations Marsden Ball
	Fixation	Marsden Ball Alphabet Fixations Wall Fixations Monocular Fixations
	Depth Perception	Brock String Convergence Stimulation Convergence Relaxation
	Peripheral Vision	Wall Fixations Brock String
	Binocular Coordination	Brock String Convergence Stimulation Convergence Relaxation
	Maintaining Attention	Rotations Marsden Ball Convergence Stimulation Convergence Relaxation
	Distance-Vision Acuity	Accommodative Rock Deep Blink

	Visualization	Palming
Running	Depth Perception	Brock String Convergence Stimulation Convergence Relaxation
	Peripheral Vision	Wall Fixations Brock String
	Distance-Vision Acuity	Accommodative Rock Deep Blink
	Visualization	Palming
	Relaxation	Palming Head Rolling Deep Blink
Dancing	Tracking	Rotations Marsden Ball
	Accommodation	Accommodative Rock Deep Blink
	Depth Perception	Brock String Convergence Stimulation Convergence Relaxation
	Peripheral Vision	Wall Fixations Brock String
	Binocular Coordination	Brock String Convergence Stimulation Convergence Relaxation
	Hand-Eye Coordination	Monocular Fixations Marsden Ball
	Maintaining Attention	Rotations Marsden Ball Convergence Stimulation Convergence Relaxation
	Visualization	Palming
Racket Sports	Tracking	Rotations Marsden Ball
	Hand-Eye Coordination	Monocular Fixations Marsden Ball
	Accommodation	Accommodative Rock Deep Blink
	Depth Perception	Brock String Convergence Stimulation Convergence Relaxation
	Peripheral Vision	Wall Fixations Brock String

	Binocular Coordination	Brock String Convergence Stimulation Convergence Relaxation
	Maintaining Attention	Rotations Marsden Ball Convergence Stimulation Convergence Relaxation
	Near-Vision Acuity	Accommodative Rock Alphabet Fixations
	Distance-Vision Acuity	Accommodative Rock Deep Blink
	Visualization	Palming
	Relaxation	Palming Head Rolling Deep Blink
Golf	Tracking	Rotations Marsden Ball
	Depth Perception	Brock String Convergence Stimulation Convergence Relaxation
	Hand-Eye Coordination	Monocular Fixations Marsden Ball
	Binocular Coordination	Brock String Convergence Stimulation Convergence Relaxation
	Maintaining Attention	Rotations Marsden Ball Convergence Stimulation Convergence Relaxation
	Distance-Vision Acuity	Accommodative Rock Deep Blink
	Visualization	Palming
	Relaxation	Palming Head Rolling Deep Blink
Swimming	Depth Perception	Brock String Convergence Stimulation Convergence Relaxation
	Peripheral Vision	Wall Fixations Brock String
	Visualization	Palming

	Relaxation	Palming Head Rolling Deep Blink
Surfing	Tracking	Rotations Marsden Ball
	Depth Perception	Brock String Convergence Stimulation Convergence Relaxation
	Peripheral Vision	Wall Fixations Brock String
	Maintaining Attention	Rotations Marsden Ball Convergence Stimulation Convergence Relaxation
	Distance-Vision Acuity	Accommodative Rock Deep Blink
	Visualization	Palming
Diving, Snorkeling	Depth Perception	Brock String Convergence Stimulation Convergence Relaxation
	Peripheral Vision	Wall Fixations Brock String
	Binocular Coordination	Brock String Convergence Stimulation Convergence Relaxation
	Maintaining Attention	Rotations Marsden Ball Convergence Stimulation Convergence Relaxation
	Distance-Vision Acuity	Accommodative Rock Deep Blink
	Visualization	Palming
	Relaxation	Palming Head Rolling Deep Blink
Sailing	Tracking	Rotations Marsden Ball
	Fixation	Marsden Ball Alphabet Fixations Wall Fixations Monocular Fixations

	Depth Perception	Brock String Convergence Stimulation Convergence Relaxation
	Peripheral Vision	Wall Fixations Brock String
	Binocular Coordination	Brock String Convergence Stimulation Convergence Relaxation
	Hand-Eye Coordination	Monocular Fixations Marsden Ball
	Maintaining Attention	Rotations Marsden Ball Convergence Stimulation Convergence Relaxation
	Distance-Vision Acuity	Accommodative Rock Deep Blink
	Visualization	Palming
Bicycling	Tracking	Rotations Marsden Ball
	Depth Perception	Brock String Convergence Stimulation Convergence Relaxation
	Peripheral Vision	Wall Fixations Brock String
	Binocular Coordination	Brock String Convergence Stimulation Convergence Relaxation
	Maintaining Attention	Rotations Marsden Ball Convergence Stimulation Convergence Relaxation
	Distance-Vision Acuity	Accommodative Rock Deep Blink
	Relaxation	Palming Head Rolling Deep Blink
Skiing	Tracking	Rotations Marsden Ball
	Depth Perception	Brock String Convergence Stimulation Convergence Relaxation

Peripheral Vision	Wall Fixations
	Brock String
Binocular Coordination	Brock String
	Convergence Stimulation
	Convergence Relaxation
Maintaining Attention	Rotations
	Marsden Ball
	Convergence Stimulation
	Convergence Relaxation
Distance-Vision Acuity	Accommodative Rock
	Deep Blink
Visualization	Palming

So, next time you think about getting in shape for the skiing season or the marathon, include your eyes in your workouts. And, don't forget about safety—not even once.

Eye Openers

• Sports and recreational activities account for more than thirty-five thousand eye injuries annually. According to the National Society to Prevent Blindness, 90 percent of all eye injuries could be avoided with proper eye protection.

• Baseball is the sport in which the largest number of eye injuries occur. In 1988 in the United States, 24 percent of sports injuries occurred during baseball games.

• Studies have shown that a racquetball traveling at about sixty-five miles per hour (about half the speed of a ball hit by good players) becomes elliptical rather than round and can therefore enter lensless eye guards. Full goggles should therefore be worn for this sport.

• Your eyes can get sunburned just as your skin can, although it may take twelve to twenty-four hours to feel the effects of the burn. Direct sunlight, reflected sunlight (on water or snow), sunlamps and welding instruments can burn the eyes.

CHAPTER 12

Eye Emergencies & Serious Conditions

From time to time, you or someone in your family will develop an eye problem that concerns or even frightens you.

For most such problems, you will want to see an eye-care professional, but it's important to know which conditions are true emergencies, which ones need prompt or immediate attention and whether you need to see an optometrist, ophthalmologist or emergency-room physician.

EYE INJURIES AND EMERGENCIES

Not all eye injuries are dire emergencies—though some are. Of course, the best way to deal with eye injuries is to prevent them from happening in the first place with appropriate safety procedures and protective eyewear. But, accidents do happen, and you should know how to recognize the kinds of problems they can cause.

In most states, optometrists can handle minor eye injuries, such as removing a foreign body that is superficially imbedded in the eye. In some states, they can prescribe certain medications, such as topical antibiotics, to treat minor eye injuries. In all states, optometrists will know ophthalmologists to whom they can refer patients with serious injuries (such as those needing surgery) and get patients seen in a hurry. So, if you think you have a serious injury but don't know any ophthalmologists, your optometrist is a good place to go to find one. Of course, if you know you have a serious injury—one involving obvious major eye damage, loss of vision or extensive bleeding—your nearest hospital emergency room is the place to go. There is really only one type of serious injury that you should try to treat before getting to an emergency room, and that is the chemical burn (see *Burns of the Eye*, page 214).

Here are some of the more common problems associated with eye injuries.

Corneal Abrasions

A *corneal abrasion* is a scraping of the cornea, most often from a foreign body—such as a grain of sand, a piece of dirt, an ill-fitting contact lens, a baby's fingernails, a twig or a mascara brush. Patients with scraped corneas will often come to the doctor saying that something is under their upper eyelid. Usually, the foreign body is no longer present, but the patient feels some discomfort as the upper eyelid passes over the damaged part of the cornea.

If you have a corneal abrasion, you may or may not feel much pain, but the eye will generally water profusely when the injury first occurs. This watering may wash out a particle that has become trapped in your eye. You can try washing out your eye with water or a commercial eyewash—*not* an "eye whitener," though. If you or someone else can see the cause of the problem (such as a speck of dirt), you can try to remove it with a clean handkerchief.

Scratches on the cornea cannot usually be seen with the naked eye. Your eye doctor will examine the injury under magnification and may also use a stain called *fluorescein* (floo-oh-RES-ee-in) to make the abrasion visible. Topical antibiotics (in the form of an ointment or drops) may be prescribed to help prevent infection. I tell my patients to get plenty of rest and take an over-the-counter pain medication if they're uncomfortable.

Doctors used to routinely patch an eye with a corneal abrasion, but many now feel the eye is better off healing without a patch. One reason is that patching an eye keeps it warmer, which increases the chance of an infection developing. Also, it's easier for a patient to monitor the eye's healing and apply mediations if the eye is not covered. On the other hand, patching is more comfortable for the patient.

Most corneal abrasions heal within a few days, although injuries from wood or other plant materials or very dirty substances may take longer.

Corneal Ulcers

A *corneal ulcer* is an open sore on the cornea and involves a deeper invasion of the corneal tissue than an abrasion. It may start with an abrasion that becomes infected, or it may start with a bacterial or viral infection that was not preceded by an injury.

Complications from contact lenses are a frequent cause of corneal ulcers today. Wearing lenses that are improperly disinfected or improperly fitted to the cornea, and leaving daily-wear lenses in while sleeping, can cause corneal ulcers. But, any injury, such as one from a twig or fingernails, can result in a corneal ulcer.

One very serious type of corneal ulcer is caused by the herpes simplex virus, which is the virus that causes cold sores and genital ulcers. A herpes infection can be transmitted to your eye if you touch a herpes sore and then touch your eye.

Most corneal ulcers are painful, and some types can be seen with the naked eye as a round depression or a white spot. Corneal ulcers caused by a herpes virus actually cause the cornea to *lose* sensitivity in the area of the ulcer, so you may not have pain as a clue that something is seriously wrong. However, the eye will be red, and you will notice a sensitivity to light. Your vision will also be blurred in the affected eye, but this is hard to notice unless the unaffected eye is temporarily covered for some reason. Under magnification, an ulcer from a herpes virus has a distinctive branching pattern, but this cannot be seen without special instruments and sometimes a fluorescein stain.

Corneal ulcers must be treated, or scarring and loss of vision can result. They are usually treated by an ophthalmologist (in some states, an optometrist may treat them) with antibiotic or antiviral medications.

If the cornea is irreparably damaged, a corneal transplant may be performed using a donor cornea (the cornea is the part of the eye that is used when eyes are donated to "eye banks"). In this procedure, the central eight to ten millimeters of the cornea are cut out. Then the new cornea is cut into the same diameter and sewn onto the eye. The thread used for this procedure is extremely thin and strong. Rejection of the donor cornea is possible, though it is not as common as with other kinds of transplants. Most corneal transplants are successful, and vision can go from extremely poor to extremely good with this type of surgery.

Cuts Around the Eye

Cuts around the outside of the eye bleed a lot and look very frightening, but they heal well, as do cuts in the conjunctiva. See your doctor if the cut is large and near the eye to be sure that no hidden damage to the eye has occurred.

Subconjunctival Hemorrhages

A *subconjunctival hemorrhage* means bleeding from broken blood vessels under the conjunctiva of the eye, between the conjunctiva and the sclera (*see* illustration, page 36 to review the anatomy and illustration, page 213).

This is a case where the problem looks much more serious than it is. Subconjunctival hemorrhages can occur with a jarring injury, such as a blow to the head from a basketball, or from anything that increases the pressure in the delicate blood vessels of the conjunctiva, such as intense coughing, sneezing or vomiting, or during childbirth. The area where the bleeding occurs appears as a bright red patch on the white sclera. There is no pain, and vision is not affected. The blood will be absorbed and the eye will return to normal within one to three weeks. Of course, if you're having any symptoms that concern you, such as pain or visual disturbances, see your eye doctor.

Hyphemas

A *hyphema* (high-FEE-mah) is a condition in which blood is sitting in the anterior chamber of the eye, in front of the iris (*see* illustration, page 213). This situation almost always arises from an injury with a blunt object; a racquetball in the eye is a high-ranking cause. You don't feel the hyphema itself, but you'll feel pain from the injury that caused it.

A hyphema is a true eye emergency, requiring immediate patching of the eye and bedrest for up to a week. Both these measures are to minimize your eye movements, promote absorption of the blood and prevent further bleeding. Without treatment, the eye may be stained with blood, resulting in permanent loss of vision. Glaucoma and a serious inflammation of the iris can also be consequences of an unsuccessfully resolved hyphema. If you suspect you have a hyphema or if you have sustained any kind of blunt injury to your eye, you should see an ophthalmologist right away. Have someone drive you to the doctor, taking care not to make any excessive head or eye movements en route.

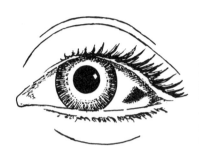

Subconjunctival Hemorrhage

A subconjunctival hemorrhage involves bleeding that appears as a bright red patch on the white sclera. There is no pain or interference with vision, and the eye will return to normal within one to three weeks. No treatment is necessary.

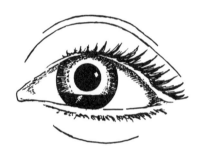

Hyphema

In this dangerous situation, blood is sitting in front of the iris. Staining of the eye and other serious problems can result from a hyphema. You should get to an ophthalmologist right away, taking care not to make any excessive head or eye movements in the meantime.

Retinal Detachment

A *retinal detachment* is the peeling away of the retina from the back of the eye, the way you might imagine wallpaper peeling away from a curved surface. The retina detaches when a hole or tear in it allows fluid to collect between it and the back of the eye, causing a separation similar to that caused by water when it gets behind wallpaper.

Retinal detachments can occur for many reasons, not all of them injuries, although a blunt or penetrating injury to the eye is a common cause of this problem. Nearsighted eyes and prominent eyes are more prone to retinal detachment, probably because their retinas are more tautly stretched. Recent cataract surgery is another risk factor.

The retina can be reattached by an ophthalmologist if the patient is seen in time. If there is only a small hole, a laser may be used to seal it. If there is a large tear and the retina is actually peeling away from the eye, a freezing probe is used to make it adhere to the eye again.

Everyone should know the symptoms of retinal detachment because failure to seek treatment in time can result in blindness in the affected eye.

A developing retinal detachment is heralded by flashes of light that look like sparks or flickers, large numbers of floaters in the field of vision and a "shadow" or "curtain" that spreads from the edge of the visual field to the central vision. A "shimmering" effect—like looking through gelatin—may also be noticed in the visual field. There is no pain arising from the retina itself because the retina does not contain pain receptors. (You may, of course, feel pain from elsewhere in the eye if an injury has caused the detachment.)

Burns of the Eye

Since the blink reflex is one of the fastest reflexes we have, the eye is rarely burned by fire. Most eye burns are caused by chemicals or by radiation of various kinds.

Chemical burns fall into the category of *acid* or *alkali* burns. Acid substances that burn the eyes include battery acid (such as that used in car batteries), industrial chemicals and liquid bleach. Alkali burns are most often caused by lye-based drain cleaners. These substances can be splashed into unprotected eyes and do a great deal of damage in a short time. Alkali burns are a lot worse than acid burns. Acid "eats through" the eye more slowly than alkali chemicals and can more often be washed out before it does any major damage.

Speed is crucial with a chemical burn. Wash out the eye with anything available—preferably water, but even milk, tea or soda will do if it has to. Hold the eye open under running water for fifteen to twenty minutes or submerge the eyes in a bucket of water. Then get to an emergency room.

The doctor will probably complete the irrigation of the eye and use an antibiotic ointment as well as give you medications to reduce inflammation and pain. The eye will be closed and patched under pressure to relieve pain and allow healing to occur.   The other type of burn that affects the eyes is a radiation burn. Radiation burns can come from too much exposure to radiation; ultraviolet, infrared, nuclear and X-ray radiation can all burn the eye.

As with other accidents, the best approach is prevention. **Never stare directly at the sun even as it is reflected on glass or water or even during an eclipse.** You can permanently damage your retinas and cause complete loss of your central vision this way. When I was a Navy optometrist, one young sailor thought he could get an easy discharge by causing himself some minor eye damage from staring at the sun. He ended up nearly blind, although he did get his discharge—a psychiatric one.

Wear appropriate eye protection if you work around excessive ultraviolet, infrared or any other kind of radiation. Be sure to wear opaque goggles if you indulge in sunbathing (which is also a skin cancer risk) under natural sunlight or in a tanning booth.

A radiation burn will leave the eyes feeling gritty and watering profusely for several hours after the exposure to the source of the radiation. You may experience a spasm of the eyelid muscles so that it is difficult to open your eyes. The eyes will be sensitive to light. Medical care consists of pain medication, bedrest, cold compresses on the eyes and topical antibiotics.

FIRST AID FOR EYE INJURIES

You should see an eye-care professional for almost any eye injury that involes swelling or bleeding and certainly for any injury that alters your vision. In the meantime, **if an eye as been injured with a blunt object and is swollen shut, do not press on the eye.** If the eye is more seriously injured than you think, you can actually squash it like a grape by pressing on it. Leave the probing to the professionals.

After you've seen the doctor, there's a first-aid principle for all injuries that also applies to the eyes, and you can use it at home. The principle is "ice the first day and heat the next." For most eye injuries, I'd modify that to: ice the first day or so until the swelling goes down, and then heat. For a bruising injury with a blunt object—otherwise known as a "black eye"— an ice bag or cold compress should be applied for the first twenty-four hours following the injury. This will help constrict the damaged blood vessels in and around the eye and reduce further bleeding and swelling. (The idea of applying a steak to the injured eye was probably just because it was cold.) The next day (and for a few subsequent days, if desired), you should apply heat to the eye. The heat causes the blood vessels to dilate (open) and absorb the fluid that is causing the swelling; the dilated blood vessels also bring in infection-fighting cells from elsewhere in the body. One way to make a hot compress for the eye that stays hot is to boil an egg and then wrap it in a towel and hold it against your eye.

Injuries that penetrate the eye—from knives, forks, scissors, pencils and toys, for example—are extremely serious and require immediate medical attention. In the meantime, you should: Cover the eye with a sterile dressing or a clean pad or cloth; not put anything in the eye; apply pressure to the forehead or cheek to stop bleeding, but do not apply pressure to the eye itself. Infection is a serious complication of penetrating eye injuries from things like scissors and pencils. Tiny fragments of metal from high-speed machinery may enter the eye and not cause much distress. If they are very hot, they may be sterile and therefore not cause an infection. However, if left in the eye, these pieces can cause a severe reaction that can even lead to blindness. So, see your doctor if you even suspect that anything has penetrated your eyeball—and wear goggles next time.

If the bones around the eyes are crushed or pushed out of alignment, they can press on the nerves or muscles around the eyes and affect vision so that you see double or have some other bizarre visual effect. **Injuries to the bones around the eyes need immediate medical attention. In the meantime, immobilize the patient's head to avoid further damage.** It's important not to panic in this situation; just get the person to an emergency room where a surgeon can quickly repair the damage.

EYE INFLAMMATIONS AND INFECTIONS

The term *inflammation* describes the response of the body's tissues to any kind of injury—whether the injury is from a poke in the eye, a disease or an allergy. It is not the same as the term *infection*, although a lot of people confuse the two words. An inflammation or "inflammatory reaction" is characterized by redness, swelling, heat (the affected area feels hot) and pain, as well as impaired functioning of the affected area. For centuries, medical students have memorized this well-recognized group of signs with the Latin words "rubor," "tumor," "calor" and "dolor"—for redness, swelling, heat and pain, respectively.

An inflammation is the body's attempt to defend itself against an invading organism (such as a virus or bacterium) or other substance (such as a piece of wood). Inflammation also occurs in other circumstances, such as during an allergic reaction. Usually, inflammation is good; it's the first step in the healing process. But, sometimes inflammations don't do any good or get out of hand and have to be controlled with anti-inflammatory drugs like steroids. When you see the suffix "itis" combined with the name for any part of the body, you can be certain an inflammation is being described.

The term *infection* describes a condition in which the body or a part of it is invaded by an organism, such as a bacterium, virus or fungus, that multiplies and produces injurious effects. An infection that is localized in a certain area of the body is usually accompanied by inflammation (the body's attempt to surround and control the invading organism), but inflammation can occur without any infection being present.

Localized infections on any part of the body (an infected finger, mouth or genitals, for example) can be transmitted to the eyes by contaminated fingers, towels or bandages. Likewise, infections of the eye can be transmitted to other parts of the body, particularly where there is an open cut or scratch. Be sure to wash your hands carefully after handling an infected eye or other body part, and wash contaiminated towels and other materials after each use.

With all that in mind, let's look at some eye inflammations and infections.

Styes

A *stye* is a common problem caused by an infection in one of the small glands on the edges of the eyelids or just under the eyelids (*see* illustration, page 218). Children frequently get styes from rubbing their eyes with dirty hands, but everyone gets one from time to time, and sometimes it's hard to say how the infection got started.

A stye looks and feels like a pimple on the eyelid—and that's really what it is. It is somewhat painful. The "pimple" can be brought to a head by steaming it. One way to do this "steam bathing" is to cover a wooden spoon with gauze and then dip the spoon into boiling water; then hold the spoon so that the steam rises to the eye but *do not touch the eye with the spoon.* Repeat the procedure as the spoon cools. Most styes go away with a week or so, but a stubborn one can be incised and drained by a doctor. Topical antibiotics are also sometimes used.

There are some over-the-counter remedies for styes that contain a compound called mercuric oxide. These remedies may work, but the mercury in these preparations can be very irritating to the eye; it causes itching, stinging and redness in many people. For this reason, I don't recommend these products.

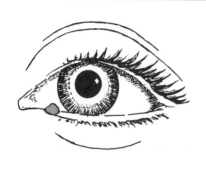

Stye

A stye is an infection in one of the small glands on the edges of the eyelids or just under the eyelid. It looks and feels like a pimple. Though a stye is not serious, it can be painful.

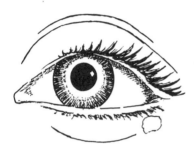

Chalazion

A chalazion results from the plugging of glands in the eyelids. It is larger than a stye and is located at some distance from the lid margin. Chalazia are not painful.

Chalazia

A *chalazion* (ka-LAY-zee-ohn) is the next step up from a stye in seriousness. (The word comes from the Greek word for hailstone. "Chalazion" is the singular and "chalazia" the plural form.) A chalazion results from the plugging of some glands in the eyelids known as *meibonian glands*, and chalazia are therefore also known as *meibomian cysts*. Under normal circumstances, the meibomian glands, which number twenty or thirty in each eyelid, secrete an oily substance that delays the evaporation of the tears and prevents drying of the eyes. Sometimes one or more of them gets plugged, and the resulting blockage causes the swelling known as a chalazion (*see* illustration above). The reason for the plugging is usually some kind of infection that makes the oily fluid thicker than it normally would be.

Chalazia are larger than styes and are located at some distance from the lid margin. They're not painful. If you're not sure whether you have a stye or a chalazion, pull the skin of the eyelid near the bump. If the skin moves and the bump doesn't, you have a chalazion. If the bump moves with the skin, you've probably got a stye.

Chalazia may occasionally grow large enough to obscure vision, at which point they can be opened and drained by a doctor under local anesthesia. A small chalazion may disappear by itself within six to eight weeks and can be helped by steam bathing, as you would do for a stye.

Dacryocystitis

The inflammation known as *dacryocystitis* (dak-ree-oh-sis-TYE-tis) results from prolonged obstruction of the tear drainage system. It's common in babies. The tears normally drain into a sac called the *lacrimal sac* that is located alongside the nose. This sac can become plugged as a result of an infection, injury, tumor or just because it's too narrow (often the problem with babies). The eye then waters profusely, and there is redness and swelling in the area of the sac (*see* illustration, page 220). The swelling may also extend to the eyelids and conjunctiva. It hurts to touch the area of the lacrimal sac.

The aims of treatment for dacryocystitis are to reopen the tear drainage system and to get rid of any infection that is causing the problem or is associated with it. Using hot compresses on the area alongside the nose and massaging the area may help open the drainage system. If necessary, a doctor can insert a probe into the lacrimal sac to open it, or minor surgery can be done. Infection is brought under control by the use of topical or systemic antibiotics (by injection or by mouth).

Conjunctivitis

The term *conjunctivitis* refers to an inflammation of the conjunctiva (*see* illustration, page 36 to locate the conjunctiva and illustration, page 220). The conjunctiva is a mucous membrane that lines the eyelids and also covers the exposed surface of the sclera.

Conjunctivitis can be caused by a bacterial, viral or fungal infection, by an allergy or by anything that has irritated the conjunctiva. When conjunctivitis is caused by an infection, it is highly contagious. You can get infectious conjunctivitis (or "pinkeye," as it's commonly called) from sharing a towel, handkerchief or makeup brush with an infected person.

You can try treating conjunctivitis with hot compresses (very warm water on a washcloth) two or three times a day. However,

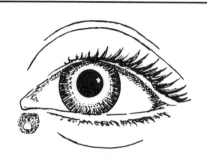

Dacryocystitis

Dacryocystitis results from prolonged obstruction of the tear drainage system. The area alongside the nose becomes red, swollen and painful to the touch, and the eye waters profusely. The swelling sometimes extends to the eyelids and conjunctiva.

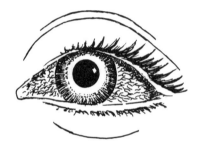

Conjunctivitis

Conjunctivitis (sometimes called "pinkeye") is an inflammation of the conjunctiva, the membrane that lines the eyelids and covers the exposed surface of the sclera. The eye looks red because of distended blood vessels over the sclera. The inner surfaces of the eyelids are also red in most cases of conjunctivitis, although in cases due to allergy, the insides of the eyelids are pale. A sticky, pus-filled discharge is characteristic of the bacterial kind of conjunctivitis. A watery discharge is more characteristic of viral and allergic conjunctivitis.

if the condition doesn't resolve within a few days, you should see a doctor because you may need an antibiotic ointment or drops if you have a stubborn bacterial infection. Don't use over-the-counter preparations that promise to remove redness from the eyes to treat conjunctivitis.

Bacterial conjunctivitis: Bacterial conjunctivitis can be recognized by a discharge with pus in it and sticky, crusty eyelids that may have to be pried open in the morning. The area under the eyelids is beefy red, and the eyes feel sore. The white part of the eye looks red with distended blood vessels. This kind of infection can happen at any age, but it's especially common in children, whose handwashing and other hygienic practices tend to be less than adequate. Children should be encouraged not to rub their eyes with dirty fingers. You can try using hot compresses to treat this condition, but you should see an eye doctor if it doesn't resolve within a few days.

Viral conjunctivitis: A viral conjunctivitis looks a little different from a bacterial one. This type is somewhat more common in adults than in children, although children also get it. This kind of infection may start in the eyes, or it may not start in the eyes at all, but may instead go along with a systemic virus that is also causing a cold or sore throat. (When this happens, it means the virus has just gotten into the conjunctiva as well as other parts of the body.) The discharge from the eyes is usually more watery and less sticky than in a bacterial infection. The conjunctiva inside the eyelids is red and sometimes has raised spots that look like little cobblestones. The eyes hurt and look red. Antibiotics won't help viral conjunctivitis, but it usually clears up within a few days without any treatment. Some doctors advise steroid ointments or eye drops to alleviate the inflammation in a viral conjunctivitis, but there's a real danger in doing this. If the infection happens to be caused by a herpes virus, the steroids can make it a lot worse. So, be careful: Sometimes it's best to just leave well enough alone.

Fungal conjunctivitis: Fungal infections of the conjunctiva can occur, especially in people whose immune systems are not functioning properly—such as cancer patients, AIDS patients and people taking drugs that suppress their immune systems (for example, after an organ transplant). These infections can be dangerous and require prompt treatment with special antifungal medications. It's hard to diagnose a fungal conjunctivitis by yourself, but if you develop any kind of conjunctival infection while on medications that suppress your immunity or while being treated for AIDS or cancer, see your doctor immediately.

Allergic conjunctivitis: As you may have guessed, allergic conjunctivitis is a conjunctivitis caused by an allergy. An important feature that distinguishes allergic from infectious conjunctivitis is *itching*. Infections of the conjunctiva hurt; allergic reactions itch. Also, the eyelashes are usually not matted with an allergic conjunctivitis as they may be with an infection, especially a bacterial one. The conjunctiva is usually swollen, and although the sclera may be red, the insides of the eyelids are pale. There is a watery discharge. Allergic reactions involving

Trachoma— A World Health Problem

An infectious conjunctivitis called *trachoma* (tray-KOH-mah) affects about four hundred million people around the world, mostly in Asia and Africa, although it is also seen in the southwestern part of the United States. It is caused by an organism that is closely related to bacteria, but it is not, strictly speaking, a bacterium. This is an extremely serious infection, which, if it is not promptly treated with antibiotics, can cause blindness.

the eyes frequently also involve sneezing, wheezing and other symptoms of allergies to animals and plants. These reactions can be treated with antihistamines by mouth or with eye drops that block allergic reactions. It's also very helpful to wash out your eyes with an eyewash if you've been around something to which you're allergic.

Conjunctivitis can be a very trivial or a potentially serious problem. See your eye doctor if your conjunctivitis doesn't clear up within a couple of days.

Blepharitis

The inflammation known as *blepharitis* (blef-ar-EYE-tis) comes from the Greek word for eyelid, which is "blepharon," and the "itis" suffix. Yes—it means inflammation of the eyelids.

In blepharitis, the tiny glands and hair follicles that open onto the surface of the eyelids become inflamed (*see* illustration, page 223). The eyelids are red, sore and sticky. There may be little ulcers on the eyelids, and some eyelashes may fall out. Styes, chalazia and dandruff of the scalp often occur along with blepharitis.

The cause of blepharitis is usually a bacterial infection when you can see ulceration (open sores) of the eyelid skin. This type needs prompt treatment with topical antibiotics. Warm compresses or scrubbing the eyelids with a special solution may also be advised.

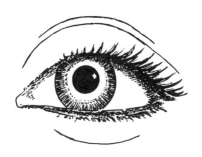

Blepharitis

Blepharitis is an inflammation of the eyelids. The tiny glands and hair follicles that open onto the surface of the eyelids become inflamed, and the eyelids are red, sore and sticky. Eyelashes may fall out.

Another cause for blepharitis is a waxy, greasy form of dandruff that affects the scalp and can also involve the eyelids, eyebrows, external ears and the area around the nose and lips. If this is the reason for the blepharitis, you may be instructed to scrub your eyelids frequently, using a washcloth or cotton-tipped applicator dipped in a solution of warm water and baby shampoo. This treatment will remove the crusty material and mucus from the eyelids. An anti-dandruff shampoo is usually recommended to bring the scalp condition under control.

Blepharitis can also be caused by exposure to dust, smoke, irritating chemicals or an allergy. Antibiotics won't help in these situations, but you can use warm soaks, remove yourself from an irritating environment and seek your doctor's advice about anti-inflammatory medications.

Iritis

An inflammation of the iris is known as *iritis* (eye-RYE-tis). This problem is characterized by a deep, aching pain in the eye and a marked sensitivity to light. There is usually a lot of watery tearing of the eye and redness around the iris, and vision becomes hazy. The pupil of the affected eye (sometimes one eye is affected and sometimes both, depending on the cause of the problem) may appear to be slightly constricted because the iris isn't reacting normally (*see* illustration, page 224). After the inflammation has been present for a while, the pupil may assume an irregular shape.

Iritis is often seen as part of a systemic disease that is characterized by inflammation of many parts of the body; diseases like lupus erythematosus and rheumatoid arthritis are in this

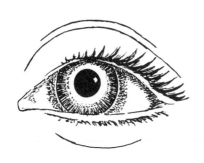

Iritis

Iritis is an inflammation of the iris. There is redness around the iris and a lot of watery tearing of the eye. The pupil may appear to be slightly constricted at first and later may assume an irregular shape. The patient experiences a deep, aching pain in the eye, a marked sensitivity to light and hazy vision.

category. It can also be caused by an infection that starts in the eye (in the cornea, for example) or elsewhere in the body, or by an injury.

This condition should be treated promptly, especially if it results from an infection. An infectious iritis can travel from the iris to the back of the eye via the choroid (*see* illustration, page 36) and do a great deal of damage. Topical and systemic steroids and antibiotics are used in treatment of this condition.

DISEASES THAT AFFECT THE EYES

There are many diseases that affect the body as a whole, including the eyes. Any systemic disease or condition that affects the nerves, muscles or blood vessels of the body is likely to have some effect on the eyes and on vision. We'll look at a few of these problems and at one problem that is strictly an eye disease. For more information about eye diseases that affect older people, such as cataracts and glaucoma, *see* chapter 5.

Retinitis Pigmentosa

Retinitis pigmentosa is a condition that causes deterioration of the retina with progressive loss of sight starting at about the age of ten. (Of all the diseases we're discussing here, this is the only one that is strictly an eye disease.) The first symptoms are increasing night blindness and difficulty seeing in dim light. Peripheral vision is then gradually lost, until the person feels as if he or she is looking through a tunnel, with only a small "island" of central vision. Fortunately, this island may last until the person is well along in years.

There is very little that can be done at this time for retinitis pigmentosa. Getting in touch with a low-vision clinic in your area and using the best low-vision aids you can obtain can help.

Diabetes

Diabetes—the medical term is *diabetes mellitus*—is a disorder of carbohydrate metabolism. The diabetic's body is unable to produce enough insulin or in some cases is unable to use the insulin it produces, which causes sugar (glucose) to stay in the blood instead of entering the cells of the body, where it is needed. Diabetes is controlled with diet and injections of insulin to create normal levels of blood sugar and normal utilization of sugar by the body's cells. For reasons that are not completely understood, diabetes also affects the blood vessels, especially in the kidneys and the eyes, even if blood sugar is being regulated and the missing insulin is being replaced.

Early in the diabetes, before blood sugar is brought under control, the diabetic will often experience blurred vision. This is because the high blood sugar causes changes in the eye's lens. Blurred vision may, in fact, be the first sign of diabetes. After an insulin dosage is determined and the disease is stabilized, the blurred vision from these lens changes will resolve, although it may recur if blood sugar rises again at any time.

After someone has had diabetes for ten or fifteen years, a more serious complication, known as diabetic retinopathy (see *Nutritional Therapy for Eye Disorders*, page 171), often occurs. Diabetic retinopathy involves dilated blood vessels and small hemorrhages of the blood vessels of the retina. These can occur without any symptoms for the patient unless they affect the macula (the area for central vision). If the macula is affected, you may see spots or streaks in your vision that correspond to the leaking blood vessels on the retina.

If you have diabetes, you should be checked regularly by an ophthalmologist. The hemorrhages of diabetic retinopathy can be coagulated with a laser. This is a painless, outpatient procedure that takes about half an hour. A medical laser is directed at the retina, where it does "spot welding" of the hemorrhages. The laser administers several hundred to a thousand flashes of light to the affected eye. You don't need any anesthesia, although your eyes will be dilated by drops, and you may feel somewhat "dazzled" for a while afterwards.

There is evidence that staying in good diabetic control—meaning keeping blood sugar normal with diet and insulin—

will minimize the long-term, as well as the short-term, complications of the diabetes.

Gonorrhea

Gonorrhea is a sexually transmitted bacterial disease that affects the genital tract and can cause blindness if it gets into the eyes. If a mother carries the bacteria in her vagina, they can infect a baby that is born vaginally and cause the baby to become blind. This is the reason for routine installation of prophylactic eye drops or ointment to newborns in hospital nurseries.

If you suspect that you or a sex partner may have gonorrhea, avoid touching your eyes with fingers that may have touched the infected area. And, of course, see your doctor to have this infection treated immediately.

Multiple Sclerosis

Multiple sclerosis is an inflammatory disease of the body's central nervous system. This disease process, which may, it is now believed, originate with a viral infection, destroys the sheaths of the body's nerves. The result is similar to what would happen if you removed the insulation from wiring; electrical impulses do not get where they're going very well and also escape into the wrong places.

Multiple sclerosis can affect the optic nerve itself, causing poor vision ranging from mild symptoms to blindness, blind spots in one's vision and changes in color vision. It can also affect the nerves that control the muscles of the eyes, causing double vision from strabismus, poor binocular coordination and an uncontrollable jerking of the eye muscles.

Fortunately, most people with multiple sclerosis have periods of remission when their symptoms get better or even disappear completely. Many years can go by before serious impairment of vision occurs—and it doesn't occur at all in some patients. Systemic steroids and other medications are used now to improve the symptoms of multiple sclerosis, including the eye problems. If you have this disease, you should see an ophthalmologist in addition to your regular doctor.

AIDS

The main eye problem for AIDS (acquired immune deficiency syndrome) patients is a greatly increased susceptibility to infections of every kind. Eye infections in AIDS patients should be diagnosed carefully and treated quickly and vigorously with the right antibiotic. The retinas of AIDS patients may also show signs of inflammation, although there are usually no visual symptoms from this problem. If you have AIDS and are having eye pain, signs of inflammation or difficulty seeing, see your doctor immediately.

OTHER CONDITIONS AFFECTING EYES

Here are some other conditions (they're not really "diseases") that can affect the eyes.

Thyroid Dysfunction

The *thyroid gland* is located in the neck. It secretes *thyroid hormones* that regulate the body's metabolic rate—the rate at which we utilize nutrients for fuel. When the thyroid gland becomes overactive and secretes too much of the thyroid hormones, the eyes are severely affected. (The actual damage to the eyes, it is now believed, may be caused not by the thyroid hormones themselves, but by antibodies to the thyroid gland, which are at the same time causing the excessive secretion of the thyroid hormones.)

With thyroid dysfunction, tissues behind the eyes swell so that the eye muscles weaken from being stretched. The eyes may cross and see double. The eyes bulge out (more of the whites show than is normal) because of the swollen tissues. And, there may be a dry, gritty feeling in the eyes, as well as redness.

The cause of the thyroid problem should be treated, but this unfortunately doesn't always solve the eye problems that the excess thyroid hormones (and possibly other substances) have caused. Further treatment, such as exercises or even surgery, may be necessary to correct these problems. The muscle problems can be corrected with surgery that tightens the muscles. The eye protrusion can be partially corrected by suturing together the outer thirds of the upper and lower lids. If the optic nerve has been compressed by the swollen tissues behind the eyes, surgery may have to be done to relieve this pressure. Patching is sometimes done during treatment, and steroids may also be used.

Migraine Headaches

The term *migraine headache* is applied to severe headaches that usually occur on one side of the head and are usually accompanied by disordered vision with nausea and vomiting. They are generally believed to be caused by dilation of arteries in the head.

It's hard to say whether a migraine affects the eyes or the eyes affect a migraine, but migraines seem to involve the eyes in some way. People with migraines report bizarre disturbances of vision during or just before the headache. Zigzags of light, double vision, flashing lights, colored lights and having half the visual field obscured can all occur. These are all temporary (they go away by the time the headache is over, which is usually a matter of hours) and are probably caused by irregular blood flow to the visual cortex in the brain.

Pain medication, medications to constrict the blood vessels and rest in a dark room are the treatments for migraines. It's important to be sure the visual symptoms go away after each episode of headache to distinguish migraine-associated symptoms from other problems involving the retina, optic nerve or other areas of the visual pathway.

Strokes and Tumors

Anything that impairs the blood supply to the optic nerve or visual pathway in the brain, or presses on the optic nerve itself, will cause marked visual disturbance. Therefore, *strokes*, which can be defined as disruptions of the blood supply to any part of the brain, and brain tumors, which can compromise the blood supply and press on structures in the brain, can cause a variety of visual symptoms ranging from slightly blurred vision to complete blindness. Unless the optic nerve or other structures have been irreparably damaged, vision usually improves after a stroke resolves or a tumor is removed.

DRUGS THAT AFFECT EYES

If diseases that affect the whole body can affect the eyes, it makes sense that medications for the whole body can also affect the eyes—and many of them do. Here are some of the more dramatic examples.

Antihistamines (brand names Benadryl, Chlor-Trimeton, Dimetane and others): Antihistamines are used in the treatment of allergic reactions and are available as oral medications and as eye drops. They cause an increase in pressure in the eye and should not be used by people who have glaucoma.

Chlorothiazide (brand name Diuril): Chlorothiazide is another diuretic that can cause blurred vision and dryness in the eyes.

Chlorpromazine (brand name Thorazine): Chlorpromazine is used in the treatment of mental disorders. It can cause blurred vision due to changes in the retina, cornea and lens.

Digoxin (brand name Lanoxin): Digoxin is used in the treatment of heart problems. It can cause a distortion of vision so that everything has a yellowish tint and can also cause blurred vision.

Ethambutol (brand name Myambutol): Ethambutol is used in the treatment of tuberculosis. It can cause a dramatic loss of vision by affecting the optic nerve behind the eyeball. It can also alter color perception.

Furosemide (brand name Lasix): Furosemide is a diuretic, or "water pill," that promotes excretion of fluid from the body. It can cause blurred vision and dryness in the eyes.

Gold (brand name Myochrysine and others): Gold is used to treat rheumatoid arthritis and lupus erythematosus. The gold can settle in the cornea, where it can cause inflammation and blurred vision.

Haloperidol (brand name Haldol): Haloperidol is used to treat mental disorders. It can temporarily paralyze the eye muscles and can cause blurred vision.

Hydroxychloroquine sulfate (brand name Plaquenil): Hydroxychloroquine sulfate is a drug that is used in the treatment of rheumatoid arthritis, lupus erythematosus and malaria. It can cause a decrease in one's ability to see the color red and a distortion of the central vision so that lines that are straight look wavy, making reading difficult.

Marijuana (popular names grass, weed): Frequent smoking of marijuana can lead to alterations in depth perception.

Oral contraceptives (brand names Ovral, Demulen, Norinyl and others): Oral contraceptives, also known as "birth control pills," can cause inflammation of the optic nerve with blurred vision and an enlarged blind spot, occlusion of the central vein in the retina, migraine headaches and poor tolerance for contact lenses.

Steroids (brand names Prednisone, Deltasone, Decadron and others): Steroids are used to treat a wide range of inflammatory conditions, including many eye conditions. They are available as oral medications, injections and eye drops. If used in high dosages for long periods of time, the oral steroids and the eye drops can cause cataracts and glaucoma. Systemic steroids can cause swelling of the optic nerve, with potential loss of visual acuity and color perception.

Tetracycline (brand name Tetracyn): Tetracycline is an antibiotic used to treat many kinds of infections, such as genitourinary infections and bronchitis. It is also used in the treatment of acne. It can cause a swelling of the optic nerve with compromise in visual acuity and altered color vision. It can also cause a burning sensation in the eyes.

Thioridazine (brand name Mellaril): Thioridazine is used in the treatment of mental disorders. It can cause pigmentation (coloration) of the retina, which may or may not affect vision.

TROUBLESHOOTING— EYE SYMPTOMS AND SIGNS

As we've seen so far, any particular symptom or sign can arise from a large number of different causes. (Doctors make a distinction beteen symptoms and signs. A "symptom" is something that can only be noted by the person who experiences it—like pain; a "sign" can be observed by an outsider—redness, for example.) Here are some symptoms and signs that can help you make a preliminary guess at what your problem might be. In most cases, you'll then want to get to your optometrist or ophthalmologist for further diagnosis.

Wet Eyes

The eyes naturally tear (water) profusely when they are irritated by anything, such as an eyelash, a speck of dirt, smoke or a cut onion. They also tear when strong emotions overtake us. When such tearing occurs for no apparent reason in one or both eyes, it may indicate a blockage in the tear drainage system (see *Dacryocystitis*, page 219), and you should see your eye doctor about it.

Dry Eyes

Eyes that are too dry are a more serious problem than eyes that are too wet because the cornea needs to stay wet to stay healthy. The eyes produce mucus if there aren't enough tears, and the eyes feel gritty, sticky and uncomfortable, and vision is poor. Dry eyes tend to occur more often as people get older and their tear production decreases. Contact lens wearers are also prone to dry eyes. If the cause of the problem cannot be corrected, artificial tears in the form of eye drops can be used. See your doctor about this condition.

Discharge from the Eyes

Discharges from the eyes are generally of two types: the watery type and the sticky type.

The watery type usually indicates one of the following: that something is irritating the eye (such as a speck of dirt or an eyelash); that the tear drainage system has become blocked; that you have a viral infection; or that you have an allergy. You may have to do a little detective work if you're not sure what's causing the problem. Do your eyes only water at certain times or in certain places—such as around a pet or while burning leaves? Is the watering associated with a cold or sore throat? If a watery discharge persists without a known and remediable cause, see your doctor.

The sticky type of discharge is sticky because of the mucus or pus that it contains. A sticky discharge that causes the eyelashes to become matted may be due to bacterial conjunctivitis (see *Conjunctivitis*, page 219) or to insufficient tear production. See your doctor if it persists.

Swelling on the Eyelids

A swelling on the eyelids is usually due to a stye or chalazion (see *Styes*, page 217 and *Chalazia*, page 218). You can try hot compresses or steam bathing of the affected area. See your doctor if the problem does not resolve within a few days.

Swelling Around the Eyes

The area around the eyes, including the eyelids, can become filled with fluid and look puffy from a variety of different causes. Eye injuries can certainly cause this area to swell, as can infections and allergic reactions. Any condition in which excess fluid is retained in the body, such as some kidney and heart conditions, may cause swelling around the eyes after the person has been lying down for a while and the fluid settles there.

If you have this kind of eye swelling with no obvious cause, check with your doctor; sometimes the swelling is the first sign of a serious illness.

Protruding Eyes

Some people have eyes that protrude or "stick out" more than the average eyes, and there is really no problem with this condition. However, if your eyes start to protrude more than they have previously, it may indicate a problem with your thyroid gland (see *Thyroid Dysfunction*, page 227). Tumors can also cause an eye to protrude. See your doctor if there is a change in the degree of protrusion of one or both of your eyes.

Red Eyes

Red eyes can come from almost any of the eye conditions we've talked about—eye inflammations, infections and irritations of all kinds cause the blood vessels of the conjunctiva to dilate. The eyes then appear "bloodshot" or red.

If your eyes are constantly red, look for an obvious cause. If there is itching, the problem is probably an allergy to something in your environment. If there is pain, the problem is likely to be an infection. If the redness occurs only in certain situations, such as while using cleaning products or cutting onions, the redness is likely to be due to a chemical irritation. If the problem persists or you suspect an infection that needs treatment, see your eye doctor.

Yellow Eyes

The sclera may appear yellow in a condition known as *jaundice.* Jaundice is characterized by a general yellowness of the skin, the whites of the eyes, the mucous membranes and body fluids. The yellow color comes from an excess of a substance called *bilirubin* in the blood, which can occur during many different conditions, such as hepatitis, gallstones and certain malignancies. See your doctor about this problem.

Drooping Eyelids

The eyelids begin to sag along with the rest of the body as people age. Older people may notice that their eyelids have gradually become droopy. The lower lids may even begin to turn outward after the age of seventy or so.

Although the problem usually isn't serious enough to warrant correction, you can have surgery for drooping eyelids in which the muscles that are attached the the lids are tightened. This is usually done as an outpatient procedure in about thirty minutes under local anesthesia. The scar on each eyelid is very small and hardly visible, but there will be some swelling of the repaired eyelid for a while afterwards; you may even appear to have a "black eye" for a few days. The most serious complication associated with eyelid repair is that 10 to 15 percent of such surgeries end up needing readjustment with further surgery because one eyelid ends up higher than the other or looks different in some other way.

A *sudden* drooping of an upper eyelid is usually the result of a malfunctioning nerve. This can arise from a stroke or brain tumor and should be checked by a doctor promptly.

Lumps in and Around the Eye

There are a number of strange-looking lumps and bumps that can occur in and around the eye. Some are not at all dangerous, while others must be taken care of immediately.

Xanthelasma: A *xanthelasma* (zan-thel-AZ-mah), from the Greek words for "yellow plate," is a small, flat or slightly raised, yellowish tumor. There may be one or more of these, and they usually occur on the upper or lower eyelids (*see* illustration, page 234). Older people, people with diabetes and people with elevated levels of fats in their blood are more likely to get xanthelasmae. These little tumors are not harmful, but they can be removed, if desired, for cosmetic reasons.

Basal cell carcinoma: A xanthelasma must be distinguished from a type of skin cancer called *basal cell carcinoma*. These

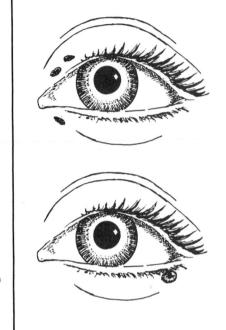

Xanthelasmae

Xanthelasmae are small, flat or slightly raised, yellowish tumors, found most frequently on the upper or lower eyelids. These tumors are harmless in and of themselves, but are associated with aging, diabetes and elevated levels of fat in the blood. They can be removed for cosmetic reasons.

Basal Cell Carcinoma

A basal cell carcinoma is a cancerous tumor of the skin, and it has to be removed. It begins as a small, shiny lump and will gradually enlarge and form a whitish border around a central depression. There may be an ulcer, which may bleed, in the central depression.

tumors begin as small, shiny lumps and gradually enlarge and form a whitish border around a central depression (*see* illustration above). There may be an ulcer in the depressed area, which may bleed. This type of cancer rarely spreads, but it definitely needs to be surgically removed. See your doctor if you're at all uncertain about what kind of lump you have.

Pinguecula: A *pinguecula* (pin-GWEK-yoo-lah, from the Latin word for fatty) is a yellowish patch that occurs in the white part of the eye, often at the "three o'clock" or "nine o'clock" position in relation to the cornea (*see* illustration, page 235). There may be several of them at a time in the eyes. (These are completely different from jaundice, which causes a generalized yellowing of the entire sclera.) Pingueculae are caused by exposure to excessive UV light, dust or wind and are common in farmers, gardeners and construction workers. They need not be removed.

Pterygium: A *pterygium* (ter-IJ-ee-um) is similar to a pinguecula, but is triangular in shape (the word comes from the Greek

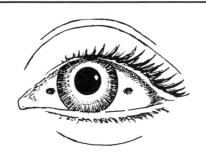

Pingueculae

Pingueculae are yellowish patches that occur in the white of the eye, most often at the "three o'clock" or "nine o'clock" position in relation to the cornea. They are caused by exposure to UV light, dust or wind. They are not considered to be harmful and need not be removed.

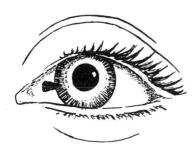

Pterygium

A pterygium looks similar to a pinguecula, but it has more blood vessels and is triangular in shape. Unlike a pinguecula, a pterygium grows into the cornea, where it can obscure vision. Pterygiums occur more frequently in hot, dusty climates. They should be removed.

word for wing) and has more blood vessels than a pinguecula. Unlike a pinguecula, a pterygium grows into the cornea, where it can obscure vision (*see* illustration above). Therefore, a pterygium should be removed. There is usually only one pterygium in the eye, and it's most often located on the side of the eye nearest the nose. No exact cause for this condition is known, but pterygiums do occur more frequently in hot, dusty climates, and I see them in my practice among surfers who spend hours sitting in the windy ocean spray and sun and get "wiped out" often. Unfortunately, these tend to grow back after having been removed.

Blurred Vision

Blurred vision is a symptom of so many different problems that some detective work and a thorough eye exam may be needed to discover the reason for it.

A frequent cause of gradually blurring vision is an increasing refractive error, causing myopia (nearsightedness) or hyperopia (farsightedness). Notice whether your blurred vision occurs when you're trying to see things at a distance or up close; then see your eye doctor for an examination to see if you need glasses or a change in your present prescription. Presbyopia, the hardening of the lens of the eye, which makes focusing difficult, can be very frightening to middle-aged people who've never worn glasses before. Some even feel they may suddenly be going blind and picture themselves tapping around with a cane. Relax— you're in good company, and the right lens prescription can usually completely correct your problem.

Visual blurring that is not due to refractive errors can be caused by a sticky discharge from the eyes, from a developing cataract or from changes in the cornea.

The cornea is very sensitive to changes in fluid balance in the body. The fluid shifts that take place during pregnancy and the menstrual cycle, as well as with high blood sugar, diabetes, heart and kidney conditions can all affect the cornea and blur vision. It's usually best to wait until a pregnancy is completed or a disease stabilized before getting a prescription for an expensive pair of glasses or contact lenses. Blurred vision can also be caused by a cornea that is developing a bulge in the center. This relatively rare condition, called *keratoconus* (ker-a-toh-KOH-nus), can only be accurately diagnosed by a doctor.

Blurred vision can also occur in glaucoma (although glaucoma usually doesn't cause any symptoms) and with a variety of other conditions and medications. Be sure to tell your eye doctor what medications you're taking when you go for your examination.

Altered Depth Perception

Inability to accurately perceive depth can occur in any condition in which vision is absent from one eye. Strabismus, amblyopia and blindness due to injury of one eye are examples of conditions that can alter depth perception. Marijuana use has also been known to cause temporary alterations in depth perception, probably by acting directly on the areas of the brain that control perception.

Loss of Central Vision

Central vision can be suddenly lost in either one or both eyes as a result of an injury to the eye or brain, a blocked artery in the retina, a hemorrhage, a stroke or a retinal detachment. These situations all either change or cut off the blood supply to the eye itself, to the optic nerve or to the visual cortex at the back of the brain.

Vision can be gradually lost due to macular degeneration (see *Macular Degeneration*, page 91), advanced glaucoma or multiple sclerosis. Vision can also be diminished by excessive smoking, lead poisoning or other kinds of poisoning, and by severe, untreated infections of the eyes, such as those caused by gonorrhea, trachoma or the herpes viruses. Diabetic retinopathy can cause loss of central vision if the blood vessels in the area of the macula are affected.

People who are losing their central vision start to perceive gaps in their vision when they are looking straight at something. For example, a book you're reading may be missing the words at the center of the page, while you can see the edges of the pages, or a face you're looking at may appear to be missing a nose.

Loss of Peripheral Vision

Glaucoma is a frequent cause of loss of peripheral vision. Unfortunately, this warning sign is not always noticed. People (or their friends) may notice that they're becoming clumsy—tripping over things and knocking things off tables—and that their driving skills have deteriorated. Such signs warrant a visual field exam with your eye doctor.

A sudden loss of peripheral vision that looks like a curtain being drawn across part of your visual field may indicate a retinal detachment and should be checked immediately.

Blind Spots

Everyone has a blind spot in the visual field of each eye (see *Blind Spots*, page 32). But, certain conditions can cause these blind spots to enlarge or cause new blind spots to occur. Glaucoma is one of these conditions, as is any kind of pressure on the optic nerve, such as that caused by a tumor. Migraine headaches can cause temporary blind spots in the visual field.

If you think you may have blind spots in your vision, make a cross in the center of a piece of graph paper and look directly at it. If parts of the graph paper are now absent or distorted in your visual field, you may have a problem and should see your eye doctor.

Missing Segments of Vision

A stroke, brain tumor or a blockage of blood vessels in the

retina for any reason can cause one-half, one-quarter or some other segment of the visual field to disappear. For example, you might be missing the upper or lower half of your normal visual field, or you might be missing the "twelve o'clock to three o'clock" segment of it. Migraine headaches can cause this phenomenon to occur temporarily.

Double Vision

Double vision—also called *diplopia* (di-PLOH-pee-ah)—means that you're seeing two objects where there is only one. The objects can be side by side, one above the other, or one can appear to be leaning to one side. A cataract can cause double (or even sometimes triple) vision in the affected eye. Double vision in both eyes can occur with high blood pressure, diabetes, a stroke or multiple sclerosis. Strabismus from any cause and eye injuries that push the eyes or eye muscles out of alignment can also cause double vision.

Flashes of Light

Flashes of light in the visual field are generally due to a retinal problem of some sort, or to migraines. The flashes can look like sparks or zigzags. When they're associated with lots of floaters, they may be a warning of impending retinal detachment. See your doctor to get an accurate assessment of your condition.

Sensitivity to Light

Sensitivity to light so that light hurts the eyes or makes them very uncomfortable can occur with certain eye conditions, such as corneal ulcers and iritis. The medical word for this symptom is *photophobia* (foh-toh-FOH-bee-ah). In the presence of ordinary light, photophobic eyes may feel the way they do when you walk out of a dark movie theater into bright sunshine.

Changes in Color Perception

As we discussed in chapter 3 (see *Color 'Blindness,'* page 41), about 8 percent of men and 0.5 percent of women have some degree of difficulty in perceiving what we think of as the "normal" range of colors. These color-deficient people have a hereditary condition, which is really no cause for concern. Some medications, such as tetracycline, hydroxychloroquine sulfate, digoxin and ethambutol (see *Drugs That Affect Eyes*, page 228) can also cause changes in color perception.

Any inflammation or damage of the optic nerve—which can be caused by a disease like multiple sclerosis or a brain tumor causing pressure in that area—can also alter color vision. Therefore, if there is no known cause for a change in your color vision, it's important to have a thorough exam. The eye doctor should test one eye at a time because color problems that exist in only one of your eyes can be compensated for by normal vision in the other eye.

Pain in the Eyes and Headaches

Pain in and around the eyes can take many forms with many different causes. If you consult a doctor about eye pain, try to describe exactly what the pain feels like (sharp, dull, deep or superficial, for example) and under what circumstances the pain occurs (after reading or using a computer, while outside in bright light and so on).

Eyestrain is a common cause for the kind of pain that feels like a muscle cramp behind the eyes and can be described as a "pulling sensation." This kind of pain frequently occurs in situations where the eyes have to accommodate for prolonged periods of time, such as while reading or using a computer. It may indicate the need for glasses, or that you need to rest your eyes more often.

A sharp but superficial pain in one eye usually indicates that something has gotten into the eye, perhaps without your being aware of it. Try to see what the problem is by looking at the sclera and under the eyelids in a mirror. If you can't easily remove the irritant, see your eye doctor.

A burning sensation in the eyes usually indicates that an irritant like smoke or a chemical (such as shampoo or the chlorine in a swimming pool) has gotten into them. You can wash your eyes with water or a commercial eyewash. It can also indicate a developing infection or inflammation in the eyes or a lack of tears in the eyes. Check with your eye doctor if the problem persists and you're not sure what's causing it.

A deep, aching pain is typical of iritis (see *Iritis*, page 223). See your eye doctor if you think you may have this condition. Sometimes, glaucoma can cause severe eye pain, but more often there are no symptoms with this disease.

A pain that seems to spread from your eyes to the area around your eyes and may involve your whole head can be caused by eyestrain, but it is often a symptom of fever or a systemic infection. Neck problems and sinus problems can also cause this kind of pain.

Headaches are often attributed to eye problems, and they can be due to refractive errors, improper lens prescriptions and problems with the muscle balance of the eyes. If your headaches occur along with reading, watching television, using a computer or some other intense use of your eyes, the problem is likely to be eye-related. However, there are many other reasons for headaches: muscle tension; intake of tobacco, caffeine or alcohol; and many kinds of illnesses, from viruses to brain tumors. An eye exam is a good place to start to diagnose your headaches, but it may not reveal the reason for them.

The signs and symptoms I've talked about in this chapter are only intended as a starting point in diagnosing an eye condition. Always see a professional if you have any questions about your eyes.

Eye Openers

• About fifty thousand Americans are the victims of home cleaning eye injuries each year.

• About one in ten thousand people is born with an absence of pigment in the eyes, skin and hair; their eyes are extremely sensitive to light, and they may also experience astigmatism and difficulty controlling their eye muscles. The condition is called *albinism* (AL-bin-izm).

• About twenty million people around the world have lost their vision to trachoma. This sad consequence of an infection can be easily prevented with antibiotics.

CHAPTER 13

Just for Fun—
Optical Illusions

We've all at one time or another been fooled by something we saw and swore was real but wasn't. Have you ever wondered how a picture hanging on a wall can appear to move, or why the harvest moon appears large and orange while the full moon at other times looks small and white? There are really hundreds of optical illusions. Some have simple explanations, some have just theories that try to explain them, and some cannot be explained. We study optical illusions because they can be tools for investigating the basic processes involved with seeing the world. But they can also be fun!

SPECIAL EFFECTS

Here are some popular illusions and the explanations that research in perception has offered to explain them. Although many of these illusions have been pondered since the nineteenth century, most of them cannot yet be entirely explained.

Necker Cube

One of the most popular illusions is called the Necker cube (*see* illustration, page 242). As you look at the cube, two images are possible. In the first, the shaded surface appears as the front of a transparent cube with the "A" in the upper righthand corner of it. In this view, the "B" appears to be on the left side of the cube in the corner farthest away from you. In the second image, the "A" appears to be on the back side of the transparent cube

Necker Cube

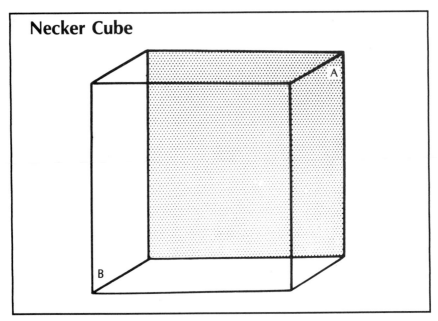

Two images are possible when you look at the Necker cube. In the first, the shaded surface appears as the front of a transparent cube with the "A" in the upper righthand corner of it. In this view, the "B" appears to be on the left side of the cube in the corner farthest away from you. In the second image, the "A" appears to be on the back side of the transparent cube (the side farthest from you), and the "B" appears to be in the near corner of the left side of the cube.

(the side farthest from you), and the "B" appears to be in the near corner of the left side of the cube.

This perception is not determined only by the lines and patterns you see; it's really your eyes and brain searching for the best interpretation from the data available. This data is the sensory information you receive as well as the previous knowledge of similar patterns. But perception goes beyond this: You assess the evidence and make the best guess. The cube has no clues as to which alternative is correct, so you'll see it first one way, then the other.

Müller-Lyer Pattern

Another popular illusion is found in the Müller-Lyer pattern (*see* illustration, page 243). This is a pair of lines of equal length, but one of them (line A in the illustration on page 243) appears to be longer than the other (line B in the illustration).

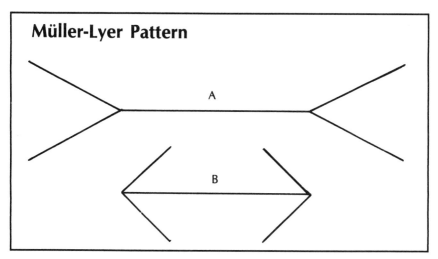

Müller-Lyer Pattern

A

B

In this illusion, line A looks longer than line B, although they are actually exactly the same length. Go ahead and measure them.

There have been many theories to explain why this illusion occurs. At first, it was suspected that the shapes at the ends of the lines forced the eyes to look in the wrong place and be deceived, but this theory doesn't seem to account for the illusion.

The phenomenon called *size constancy* may play a significant role in this illusion. Size constancy is the tendency for the perceptual system to compensate for the changes that objects appear to undergo as they are viewed from different distances. Although the image an object projects onto the retina increases in size when an object is brought closer to the eyes, you can perceive the object as the same size it was before it was moved because your brain tries to preserve "size constancy." You can try this by holding one hand up and extended at arm's length and the other hand up about halfway between your eyes and the other hand. When the hands are held up so that they don't overlap, you perceive them as being the same size (because you know they are). But, when you move the closer hand so that it overlaps the more distant hand, the closer hand appears large enough to obliterate the more distant hand (your size constancy has not been preserved here).

When you look at lines A and B in the illustration above, one way to perceive them is as parts of figures with corners. Line A can appear to be a recessed part of a figure, and line B can appear

Impossible Figure

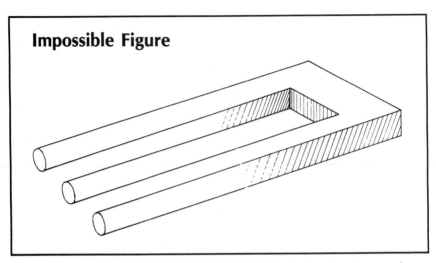

This figure presents a problem because the visual clues it gives the viewer make no sense. Are there three prongs or two? Are the prongs cylindrical or rectangular?

as a part of a figure that is bowed toward you. The brain therefore perceives line A to be more distant and line B to be closer, says the theory, and it then compensates for the difference in distance by making line A appear longer.

The Impossible Figure

The illustration above is popularly called "the impossible figure," and it may be obvious why. The problem here comes from an ambiguity as to the depth of the figure. The eye is not given the necessary information to locate the parts in space. The visual brain is an active system because it functions even if there's no reliable information. It searches out the clues and seeks to make sense of them. In this case, the lines make no logical sense, so your brain can't make up its mind!

Redundant Pattern Illusion

The figure on page 245—called a "redundant pattern"—seems the most disturbing of all! However, it is not exactly clear what is causing the effect.

One theory says that the peripheral retina, which is more sensitive to movement than the central retina, becomes overstimulated by the pattern and sends signals to the brain that indicate the figure is moving. Another theory says that the retina tries

Redundant Pattern

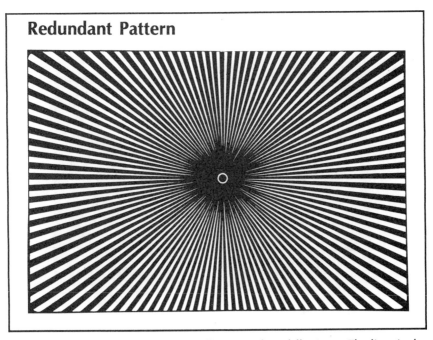

Look at the circle in the center of this illustration for a full minute. The lines in the figure will start to look wavy. Then, stare at a blank wall, and you see a pattern that looks like grains of rice swirling around.

to save itself time and energy in analyzing information by assuming that, if a portion of a pattern is redundant, then the rest of the pattern is the same. Both explanations suggest that the retina itself is responsible for the movement effect of this pattern.

Try this little experiment: Look at the central circle for about a full minute. The lines in the figure will start to look wavy. Then stare at a blank wall. You should notice movement similar to grains of rice swirling around. The aftereffect is probably the retina trying to recover from the redundant stimulation.

Two-Faced Vase

The "two-faced vase" is a famous illusion (*see* illustration, page 246). The visual problem is the lack of clues to discern which image is the "figure" and which is the "background" (called *figure-ground discrimination*). At first glance you may see two faces, facing each other. After a few seconds you may see a vase (white) against a dark background. This illusion is similar to the

Two-Faced Vase

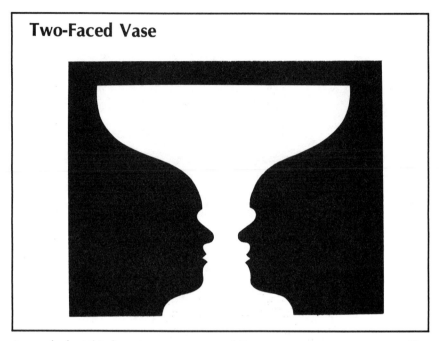

As you look at this figure, you may see a white vase—or you may see two profiles in black facing each other. There is an absence of clues as to which part of this picture is the "figure" and which is the "ground" ("background").

Necker cube in that there is an absence of clues as to how one part of the figure is oriented with respect to other parts of the figure. Very confusing!

Hermann-Hering Grid

As you look at the illustration on page 247, which is called the Hermann-Hering grid, you'll see gray areas at the white intersections. But notice that the one intersection at which you are directly looking is always white! And no matter which intersection you look at, it will always be the one that is white. The explanation for this is related to the way the retina works to enable us to see contrasts.

Here's the theory. Recall from chapter 3 that there are approximately 120 million rods and 7 million cones that converge to form only about a million nerve fibers that make up the optic nerve. Each bundle of rods and cones in one fiber is called a *retinal field*. The retina uses these retinal fields to help us distinguish patterns and contrasts in the world, such as the

Hermann-Hering Grid

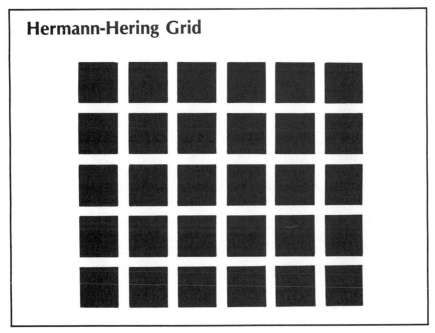

As you look at this figure, you'll see gray dots at the corners of the white intersections. But, if you focus directly on one particular white intersection, you won't see a gray dot. Move your focus to another intersection and the gray dot will reappear at the first one.

pattern in this illusion. The stimulation of one retinal field inhibits the firing of an adjacent one. While looking at this illusion, however, some areas of overlapping retinal fields are stimulated, and this phenomenon causes the apparent "shadows" at the intersections of the grid. The central retinal field is not affected, so the intersection at which you're directly looking stays white.

ILLUSIONS IN EVERYDAY LIFE

It's fun to look at some of the classic illusions like the ones on these pages, but life is full of everyday illusions that are just as interesting.

Some everyday illusions are easy to explain, while others still mystify the experts.

The Case of the Moving Incense

Here's an illusion you can do yourself. Light a stick of incense, and set it in a holder with the lit end in view. Darken the room completely, and stand at the other end of the room from where the incense is. As you watch the tiny light, it will soon appear to wander around, sometimes just swinging back and forth, occasionally darting in one direction or another. There is no actual movement, only an apparent one, which is called an *autokinetic phenomenon*.

The reason for this illusion is not as simple as one might think. Researchers studying it originally thought that the the eyes couldn't maintain their fixation on the small target with no other visual clues and that this lack of fixation caused the perception of movement, but that explanation proved to be wrong. The eye muscles *do* maintain the gaze on the small object successfully, but to do so they must constantly send "adjusting" signals to the brain. These signals are to *prevent* the eyes from moving and to keep them fixated. However, these same signals "fool" the brain into perceiving movement in the environment.

The Changing Moon

Why does the moon appear to be much larger when it is near the horizon than it does when it is directly overhead? Scientists have pondered this for many years and still don't have a good explanation.

Researchers originally thought that the apparent difference in size might be due to the elevation of people's eyes as they looked at the moon straight ahead (the horizon moon) versus looking up at an angle (the overhead moon). Experiments showed that the perceived difference in size was *partly* related to the angle of elevation of the eyes, but that this was not the whole explanation.

Another explanation suggested that the horizon moon might look larger because it can be more directly compared with objects on the ground, such as buildings and trees. But, this theory was quickly debunked when it was found that the horizon moon appears equally large over water or desert surfaces where there are no objects with which it can be compared.

The most likely explanation for this illusion is that the brain perceives the sky as a dome, the way the ancients thought the heavens were actually structured. If the sky were a dome, the moon would really be farther away when directly overhead than it would be at the horizon. So, here again, the brain may be making an interpretation that fools the eyes.

The Changing Sun

The setting sun appears much larger than the noonday sun. It is believed that, at the end of the day, heat from the earth is radiating upward so that we are viewing the sun through a warmer atmosphere, which makes it appear larger.

Oasis in the Desert

What about the illusion of an oasis in the desert or water on a hot highway? This common illusion is explained this way: On an extremely hot day, heat begins to radiate upward from the earth. The light rays from the sky enter this very hot atmosphere and cannot reach all the way to the earth before they are reflected by the heat waves. The "water" that appears on the ground is a reflection of the light rays from the sky.

Moving Lights

If you've ever been to Las Vegas or seen any of the older movie marquees, you'll recall the apparent movement of the lights as they beckon you to enter the casino or theater. These lights are not really moving, but they give the illusion of movement by making use of a visual effect called the *phi phenomenon*. The phi phenomenon says that when two lights are timed appropriately, they will give the appearance of the light moving from one location to another because the lights are stimulating adjacent areas of the retina.

Moving Pictures

If an ordinary incandescent bulb is switched on and off at a certain frequency—about thirty flashes per second—it will appear to the human eye as one continuous light. This frequency is called the *critical fusion frequency*. For very bright lights, including fluorescent lights, the critical fusion frequency is higher—about fifty flashes per second, depending on the brightness. (Fluorescent lights bother us when they get old because their flashing frequency drops below our critical fusion frequency, and we see the flickering.)

Cinema pictures are projected at twenty-four frames per second, which is well below our critical fusion frequency, and, in the early days of movies, the flicker was obvious to the viewer. Modern projectors have a special shutter that shows each picture

Eye Openers

- People have probably wondered about natural illusions since ancient times, but the scientific study of illusions only began about a century ago. It may be that the invention of optical instruments such as cameras and stereoscopes stimulated people to think more about perception. And, the invention of better writing tools in the 1850s let everybody do more doodling, which probably led to the chance discovery of many optical illusions.

- Drawings that are done "in perspective"—that is, they create the illusion of depth—are taken for granted today. But, it wasn't until the fifteenth century that artists were able to master this kind of optical illusion. A fresco painted by the artist Masaccio in Florence, Italy in 1428 is said to be the first example of convincing perspective drawing. The fresco, called "The Holy Trinity, the Virgin, St. John and Donors," seemed to dissolve a wall, revealing a hidden chamber behind it.

- In 1906, explorer Robert E. Peary wrote that he had discovered snow-capped mountains in the arctic that were at least fifteen thousand feet high, more than twice the height of any mountains known in the region. However, he was unable to traverse the distance needed to reach these mountains. Seven years later, a second arctic expedition was led by Donald B. MacMillan, who also excitedly wrote that he had seen these peaks in the distance. As he and his exploration party got closer, however, the mountains disappeared; they found only a wasteland of broken ice. This illusion is due to the atmosphere's reflection of ice and clouds back onto the snow. It's now called "Fata Morgana," after a legendary nymph who created castles in the air.

three times in rapid succession, so that the flicker rate is effectively increased to seventy-two flashes per second, well above the critical fusion frequency for most people. Modern films appear to our eyes as continuous sequences of light and movement.

Physiologists and other scientists study illusions for clues to the workings of the brain and the visual system, but illusions have probably been noted—and played with—for as long as humans have been on earth. Next time you think you can see everything exactly the way it is, take a second look. You may be surprised.

CHAPTER 14

The Future
of Eye Care

The year is 2020. You're strolling down the walkways of a shopping mall. Simulated sunlight makes everything look warm and inviting in the center of the mall, and most shoppers don't realize that the spectrum of light is slightly different in each store, according to what colors each retailer wishes to enhance. You come across a small booth in the center of the mall with a sign that says "Eye-Tron." You walk up to the booth and insert your credit card. A voice asks you to be seated, put your chin and forehead in the headrest and just look straight ahead.

You look at a picture of a tractor driving in an open field and you hear "zip, zip." Your refractive error has been determined. Next you see a picture of ocean waves and hear "brrr, brrr." The curvature of your corneas has been measured. Then a red light comes on and you hear "bzzz, bzzz" as the thickness of your corneas is recorded. The voice asks you whether you would like to order glasses or contact lenses. If you say you would, it asks you to look carefully at the target in front of you while you "try on" different eyeglass frames or different kinds of contacts. You make your selection, and the voice instructs you to return next week for a follow-up check as your receipt pops out of a slot. "Your credit card will be charged automatically," says the voice, adding, "Have a nice day!"

Sound wild? Well, maybe, but the devices and technical knowledge to do all these things are nearly available today. In fact, we may soon see a time when, under the supervision of a doctor, machines like the fictional "Eye-Tron" will be used to routinely reshape corneas, eliminating the need for corrective lenses altogether.

Of course, technology is not the only area in which we'll see tremendous progress in the next few decades. Research in basic science, neurology, computer imaging, biochemistry, ophthalmology and physiology will no doubt reveal more and more of the secrets of the visual process and help us find methods of preserving and improving it.

HIGH-TECH EYE EXAMS

Technology is changing the way we examine eyes. The immediate future promises more accurate and faster diagnostic capabilities.

Visual field testing: Just a few years ago, many optometrists and ophthalmologists tested a patient's visual fields with a black felt board and a white-tipped pointer. The patient had to indicate when he or she first saw the pointer come into view, a process fraught with both examiner and patient errors.

Today's offices are equipped with a computerized visual field tester. The patient puts her head in a drum, and lights are flashed at specific points corresponding to areas of the retina. She indicates when those flashes are noticed by pressing a button, and the computer records each button pressed. The computer then generates a printed map of the patient's visual fields and blind spots. One unit is equipped to operate by using the patient's voice instead of having her press a button. Another unit is so sensitive that it will repeat a test of a particular spot if the patient blinks, just to verify that it was not a blind area. The newer models will be more and more independent of human assistance — and less and less subject to human error.

Photographing the inside of the eye: Looking inside the eye can often be a lengthy and uncomfortable experience. It is usually easier if the eye is dilated, allowing the doctor to look inside without the pupil constricting and blocking the view. However, dilating the eye makes the patient more sensitive to light and prevents him from reading for many hours. Special cameras have been developed that can take a picture of the inside of the eye without any special drops and can develop it in one minute. They may soon replace the present method of dilation for eye exams.

Color vision testing: The traditional way to test for color deficiency is to have the patient look at colored numbers that have been imbedded in a background of different colors. The person then tells the doctor what numbers he sees. This test has been used for many years and is fairly accurate, but it only gives the doctor a rough idea of the patient's color perception. Researchers are now trying to use the brain-wave patterns that occur in response to seeing different colors to objectively determine whether a person has a color deficiency. This more accurate form of color vision testing may lead to quicker diagnosis of certain eye diseases or tumors, as well as to more understanding of the retina-brain connection regarding our processing of color and how it is perceived.

Infant eye testing: Brain waves are also being used to study the vision of infants and others who can't communicate what they are seeing. Brain waves from the visual cortex and other parts of the visual system can now be isolated from other brain waves and studied to see whether or not someone can see. In the future, these tests may be refined to the point where doctors can tell exactly how *well* a patient can see and whether the visual system is developing normally. This technology will be especially important in caring for premature infants.

Viewing the brain: Another kind of examination of the brain uses a technology called *positron emission tomography*, or *PET*, scans. In this kind of exam, which is still experimental, naturally occurring substances, such as carbon and oxygen, are made radioactive, so that their path through different parts of the brain can be followed. When and if PET scans become available, the chemical reactions in the visual system will be observable, leading to early detection of diseases, results of injuries and many other conditions that affect vision.

Help from the computer: As you might expect, the computer will be a major factor in eye examinations in the future. You'll walk into your eye doctor's office (or the mall), sit at a terminal station and insert a card with all of your personal data encoded on the back. Then you'll tell the computer your eye-related history and symptoms, probably by just talking to it. The computer will ask for any other specific information it may require, such as the date of your last eye exam. The information will then be fed into the main office computer, which will pass it into the terminal in the doctor's office. Your glasses will be read by an automated lens meter, which will also electronically transfer the prescription to the doctor's terminal. The results of your previous eye exams will be accessed by the computer as well. Your present refractive errors (myopia, hyperopia or astigmatism) will be automatically determined, as will the eyeglass prescription to correct the problem. If you desire contact lenses, the curvature of the cornea will be determined by the computer, and the lenses will automatically be ordered once the computer has determined which lens would be appropriate for your visual needs. There may also come a time when the computer will direct a laser to alter your corneas or intraocular lenses to correct your refractive error, eliminating the need for glasses or contact lenses entirely.

EYEGLASSES OF THE FUTURE

Although refractive surgery and other technologies may someday make glasses obsolete, they'll probably be around for a while—but that doesn't mean they can't be improved.

Lenses

Today, we have glass and plastic lenses. Tomorrow we'll probably improve these materials and have an additional material or two to make lenses thinner, stronger and lighter in weight. We'll also see advances in photochromic lenses and lenses for special applications.

High-index plastics and glass: New types of *high-index* plastics and glass are now being developed. The "index" of a transparent material is a measure of the density of it, indicating how fast or slowly light travels through it. A higher index means that light travels through the material more slowly relative to a lower-index material. For example, light will travel more slowly through water than it will through air, so water has a higher index than air. The higher the index of the material, the more it bends the light, so a thinner lens of higher index will bend the light as easily as a thicker lens of lower index. High-index plastic lenses will be better than polycarbonate mostly in their ability to transmit light in the higher prescriptions without the distortions often seen with polycarbonate. These lenses will also be thinner and lighter than anything previously made.

New photochromic lenses: New developments on the sunglass horizon are photochromic plastic lenses—lenses that darken in bright light and lighten in dim light. Present manufacturing techniques can only make such lenses in glass. However, many companies are working to develop a plastic lens that can change color or intensity in sunlight. One company is experimenting with *liquid crystal* technology to achieve this. The digital readings you see on watches and the screens of some computers use liquid crystals (the screens are called *liquid crystal display* or *LCD*). The liquid crystals will be laminated between two other pieces of plastic and will react to the surrounding light by reorienting themselves.

Shutter lenses: A new high-speed "shutter" lens is being researched that can change from clear to opaque in less than 1/20,000 of a second, using this same LCD technology. This would have tremendous potential to save the vision of welders and other workers who are exposed to sudden flashes of light that can injure their eyes in seconds. The lens color would clear as fast as it darkens.

Flickering lenses: Another use for LCD technology will be in preventing motion sickness and seizures. A manufacturer is looking into the possiblity of having a lens with liquid crystals that will "flicker" light at a rate that will relieve the symptoms of motion sickness. Similar lenses may be developed that can prevent seizures in people who are prone to them when they encounter light flashing at a particular frequency.

Frames

New developments in frame materials and design will continue to improve the comfort, durability and attractiveness of eyeglasses.

Carbon graphite and memory metals: A new carbon graphite material is being developed for eyeglass frames that is thin, lightweight, comfortable and not too expensive. It retains its shape and can be coated with different colors and designs. Also being tested are materials called "memory metals." These are metals that, once shaped, retain that shape regardless of any amount of twisting or distortion. One company has already released frames with such a metal; the bridge or nosepiece of the frame can be "wrung out" like a sponge and will then bounce back into shape when released. This is the frame we'll recommend for patients who say that they are tough on their glasses! Several companies are researching ways of coloring the new metals. Aside from the traditional gold and silver, new iridescent colors and "cool colors" are being designed.

Telescoping frames: New folding designs for frames are also under investigation. For hundreds of years, the temples (earpieces) of eyeglasses have folded flat against the frames for storage. But, this tends to loosen the hinges over time, and lenses can be scratched this way. A new design has the temples telescoping into the frame the way a car's antenna telescopes into the car when you want to get it out of the way.

Computer-assisted selection: The dispensary of the future will use computer imaging to aid in the fitting and selection of eyewear. Your face will be televised on a screen, and the optician will use computer-generated overlays to "put frames on." Then, when the proper shape for you is determined, different colors will be added to see which one works best with your complexion. This way, thousands of different combinations can be tried in a short time without undue wear and tear on the frames, the customer or the optician!

CONTACT LENSES OF THE FUTURE

The revolution in contact lenses has been going on for a number of years and will continue to expand. During the 1980s, new materials were developed to try to achieve the perfect combination of visual acuity, gas (oxygen and carbon dioxide) transmission, deposit resistance, comfort, ease of care and durability in contact lenses. The next few decades will provide contact lens wearers with even better materials and more options.

New materials: The 1990s are likely to provide contact lens wearers with new fluorine compounds and perhaps other materials that are even better with respect to gas transmission, wetting ability, deposit resistance, infection resistance and comfort than the present "gas-permeables." Many doctors see these new gas-permeables as the lenses of choice in the future. One company is now working in conjunction with NASA to formulate a lens material in space and see whether better materials can be made in a gravity-free atmosphere. This would really be a space-age plastic!

A new lens design now being perfected combines the best aspects of soft and gas-permeable lenses. It's designed with a gas-permeable central section and a "skirt" made of a soft-lens material around its perimeter. This lens could solve many of the problems of millions of now-unsuccessful contact lens wearers.

Contact lenses made out of collagen, a human protein, are now receiving research and development funding. What could be more natural and compatible with the human eye than protein itself?

Also under investigation is a contact lens that comes in a liquid form. This "eye drop" contact lens is intended to be placed in the eye in a liquid state, where it will gel enough to maintain a rigid shape and correct eyesight. After a short period of time, it will begin to break down and get washed away by the tears. Another drop will be required to replace it. This would be the ultimate disposable contact lens!

New colors: Colored contacts will improve in the future and will provide a more natural look to the eye of the wearer. Eventually, more companies will develop colored lenses, and most contacts will have a slight "handling" tint to allow the wearer to see the lens when it is not in the eye.

UV protection: I believe all contact lenses will eventually be designed to block out ultraviolet light because I think we're going to get confirmation that the sunlight we receive is damaging the unprotected eye.

Photochromic contacts: Once the photochromic process is perfected for plastic eyeglass lenses, it should only be a matter of time before the technology will allow manufacturers to develop a color-changing contact lens. This will again revolutionize the contact lens industry.

Computer-assisted fitting and manufacturing: Computer imaging techniques will be used routinely in the fitting of contact lenses and in color selection. Computers will determine the shape of the cornea for fitting the lenses. Then, while holding the patient's image on a screen, different lens colors can be "tried on" to see the effect of each color. Sophisticated computer programs will play an increasing role in the design and manufacturing of all contact lenses in the future.

Easier disinfection: The disinfection of contact lenses has gone through many changes in the last decade, from cumbersome heat sterilization to different methods of chemical disinfection. In the next decade, we'll probably see a microwave disinfecting system that can clean and disinfect lenses in minutes, or even seconds.

NEW EYE TREATMENTS AND SURGERIES

Today's treatments for cataracts, glaucoma, retinal detachments and many other eye conditions would have seemed futuristic fifty years ago. And, the thought of correcting refractive errors with surgery instead of glasses was science fiction. In the same way, today's futuristic experiments will be tomorrow's commonplace realities.

Refractive surgeries: The hottest topic of the 1980s in eye surgery was radial keratotomy. Now, technological advances are looking into newer and better ways to achieve the same results as radial keratotomy and other refractive surgeries with fewer risks. One area is called *corneal sculpting*. In this procedure, a computer-controlled laser is used to reshape the cornea to improve vision. Two types of lasers are being used experimentally to do corneal sculpting. One type uses ultraviolet light to shave off a layer of the outer cornea to correct its shape; the other focuses a visible green light behind the surface of the cornea and vaporizes a pocket of cells without harming the intervening tissue. These procedures show great promise, but the jury is still out on corneal sculpting—and on which kind of laser is better for the job.

In another new procedure to correct myopia, a new material that is similar to a contact lens is surgically implanted into the cornea of the patient, creating a different curvature to the cornea.

New treatment for glaucoma: Glaucoma patients may soon benefit from a new method of treatment that uses *ultrasound*—high-frequency sound waves—instead of a scalpel or a laser (*see* illustration, page 261). The sound waves create pores in the eye

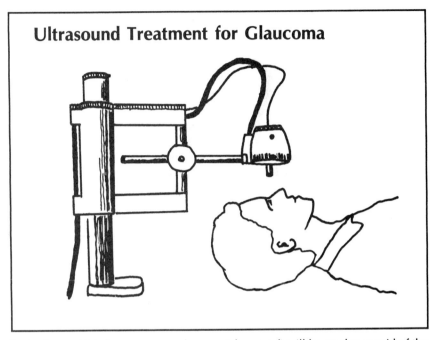

Ultrasound Treatment for Glaucoma

In the future, high-frequency sound waves (ultrasound) will be used to get rid of the excess fluid in the eye that exists in glaucoma. The sound waves will open tiny channels in the eye that allow the fluid to escape and will destroy very small sections of the eye where the fluid is being produced.

that release excess fluid and destroy very small sections of the part of the eye where the fluid is produced. The ultrasound treatment is expected to be an office procedure.

New cataract surgeries: New cataract procedures are being investigated, including one that involves only a small slit incision to insert an expandable intraocular lens that reaches its full size once inside the eye.

Other experimental procedures promise to restore focusing ability to the lenses of cataract patients. In one such procedure, a small metal pellet is injected into the lens in the patient's eye. The pellet will then be manipulated magnetically to break up the lens with the cataract, and a small needle will remove the lens particles, leaving the entire lens capsule intact. After the old lens is removed, a rubbery gel will be injected into the remaining capsule, filling it completely and allowing the muscles to once again control a clear, flexible lens within the eye.

Artificial corneas, intraocular lenses and retinas: Advances in artificial corneas, intraocular lenses and even retinas may someday routinely provide us with "spare parts" for these vital parts of the visual system.

Corneas from human donors have been used to replace damaged corneas for some time now, and there has been a good success rate with this kind of surgery. Now, artificial corneas are in the research laboratories. These corneas will probably one day be mass-produced with specified curvatures. They'll be cheaper, easier to store and more easily available than the human kind.

Artificial intraocular lenses have been used in cataract patients for many years (see *How You See After Cataract Removal*, page 88). But, these artificial lenses do not have the ability to change focus for distance or near. In the future, intraocular lenses that *can* change focus are a real possibility. One researcher is attempting to insert a lens that can be reattached to the muscles within the eye so that control of focusing can be regained. Another design involves implanting a lens that will change its shape in response to pressure, so that touching the eye through the eyelid will cause the lens to refocus.

The retina is far more complex than the cornea or lens of the eye. But, a Japanese firm has developed a prototype for an artificial retina that could someday restore sight to victims of retinitis pigmentosa, diabetic retinopathy, macular degeneration and many other conditions. The device, which transforms optical signals into electrical pulses, will first be used in computer systems and video camera lenses. Its developers believe that within a few decades such devices might be connected to the human nervous system, where they may help people with poor eyesight due to retinal problems.

NEW VISION DEVICES

People with low vision will have more options in the near future. A device now being developed jointly by NASA and the Johns Hopkins Wilmer Eye Institute is a pair of glasses in which the lenses are actually miniature TV screens (*see* illustration, page 263). The glasses, which look like mirrored sunglasses from the outside, are wired with sensors that transmit images from the glasses to a computer that is worn on the person's shoulders or waist. The computer then projects the images onto liquid crystal TV screens on the "lenses" of the glasses. Tiny

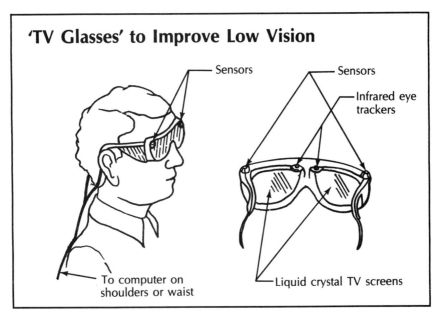

'TV Glasses' to Improve Low Vision

Sensors — Sensors

Infrared eye trackers

To computer on shoulders or waist

Liquid crystal TV screens

In the future, these glasses may enable people with very low vision to function more normally. Small sensors in the frame transmit images to a computer strapped to a person's shoulders or waist. The computer projects the images onto liquid crystal TV screens on the eyeglass lenses, while infrared trackers follow the eyes' movements so that the images move as the person's eyes move.

infrared eye trackers in the glasses keep the image moving as the eyes move.

Another area in which technology is rapidly expanding is the area of computer software and hardware for the blind and nearly blind. There are now software programs that greatly magnify the symbols that appear on computer screens for the nearly blind. For those with no vision, there are software programs that can now generate either speech or braille from documents they receive. A special printer must be used with the computer to produce the raised braille symbols.

VISION THERAPY OF THE FUTURE

Although we usually think of new computers and surgeries when we think of the future, I certainly believe there will be a place for vision therapy. Of course, some of this therapy will require some pretty fancy equipment of its own.

Eye Openers

• Computers that can be controlled by eye movements are now being developed. This technology would allow quadriplegics to dial a telephone, or leave a surgeon to control a microscope with her eyes while leaving her hands free to do surgery. The system works by using light that is reflected off the eye and keeping track of the differences between the dark and white areas.

• New antiviral drugs are being developed that may cure herpes and other viral infections that can cause serious damage to the eyes or blindness. For example, the drug ganciclovir was approved by the FDA in 1989 to treat a virus called CMV that can infect the retinas of AIDS patients and others whose immune systems are compromised.

• A new way to prevent blindness in premature infants is now under investigation. The treatment involves touching the edge of the infant's developing retina with nitrous oxide or carbon dioxide. This procedure creates scar tissue around the retina, which prevents abnormal blood vessels from growing onto the central part of the retina. The scarring seems to cause some loss of peripheral vision, while protecting the infants' more important central vision.

• Recent experiments suggest that people rapidly adapt to staying awake at night when they are exposed to very bright lights that simulate sunlight during the night. This finding is a step in helping people adapt to night shifts and international travel across time zones, but the most effective timing and duration of the light exposure has yet to be determined.

Biofeedback: The use of *biofeedback* in vision therapy may be of interest in the future. The process of biofeedback can be described as a technique for making normally unconscious or involuntary bodily processes perceptible to the senses so they can be brought under conscious control. Right now, some therapists are using an electronic device that can detect focusing movements within the eye and convert them to audible sounds. These sounds are then monitored by the patient and can be controlled by the patient's relaxing the focusing of the lens inside the eye. With training, the patient is taught how to control her own focusing and reduce eyestrain.

Alpha rhythms: The *alpha rhythm*, which is also called the *alpha wave*, is an electrical rhythm of the brain that is associated with a state of wakeful relaxation. It has a frequency of eight to thirteen cycles per second. A new vision therapy technique involves the placing of two lights over a patient's closed eyelids and having them flash at the frequency of the alpha rhythm to induce relaxation. This may be a better way to unwind from a hard day's work than sitting in front of the TV screen.

There has been rapid progress in eye care in this century, and most of us rightly expect that we will have our vision throughout our lives. It may seem to some that we have already reached the last frontier, that diseases like retinitis pigmentosa will never be curable, that blindness from brain damage cannot be challenged or that we will always have a good percentage of the population that is severely nearsighted. But, such assumptions should not be made. The next century—even the next few decades—may well provide answers to all the problems we've posed in this book and some that are yet to be uncovered.

Additional Resources

BLINDNESS AND LOW VISION

American Council of the Blind, Inc.
1211 Conneticut Ave., NW, Suite 506
Washington, DC 20036
202-833-1251

American Foundation for the Blind
15 West 16th St.
New York, NY 10011
212-620-2000
Regional Offices:
Chicago, IL   312-269-0095
Atlanta, GA   404-525-2303
Dallas, TX   214-352-7222
San Francisco, CA   415-392-4848
Washington, DC   202-492-0358

Association for the Education and Rehabilitation of the Blind and Visually Impaired
206 North Washington, Suite 320
Alexandria, VA 22314
703-548-1884

Kansys, Inc.
Computer software products and services for the blind
1016 Ohio St.
Lawrence, KS 66044
913-843-0351

National Association for the Visually Handicapped
305 East 24th St.
New York, NY 10010
212-889-3141

National Federation of the Blind
1800 Johnson St.
Baltimore, MD 21230
301-659-9314

National Society to Prevent Blindness
500 East Remington Rd.
Schaumburg, IL 60173
312-843-2020
800-331-2020

Research to Prevent Blindness, Inc.
598 Madison Ave.
New York, NY 10022
212-752-4333

DYSLEXIA AND LEARNING DISABILITIES

American Speech-Language-Hearing Association (ASHA)
10801 Rockville Pike
Rockville, MD 20852
301-897-5700

**Association for Children and Adults
with Learning Disabilities (ACLD)**
4156 Library Rd.
Pittsburgh, PA 15234
412-341-1515

Irlen Institute for Perceptual and Learning Disabilities
4425 Atlantic Ave., Suite A-14
Long Beach, CA 90807
213-422-2723

The Orton Dyslexia Society
724 York Rd.
Baltimore, MD 21204
301-296-0232

LIGHTING

Duro-Test Corporation
9 Law Drive
Fairfield, NJ 07007
201-808-1800
800-289-3876

General Electric Company Lighting Information Center
Nela Park
Cleveland, OH 44112
216-266-3900

ORTHOKERATOLOGY

National Eye Research Foundation—
International Orthokeratology Section
910 Skokie Blvd., Suite 207A
Northbrook, IL 60062
800-621-2258

SPECIFIC CONDITIONS

American Diabetes Association
P.O. Box 25757
Alexandria, VA 22313
703-549-1500
800-232-3472

Foundation for Glaucoma Research
490 Post St., Suite 1042
San Francisco, CA 94102
415-986-3162

National Multiple Sclerosis Society
205 E. 42d St.
New York, NY 10017
212-986-3240

Retinitis Pigmentosa Foundation
1401 Mt. Royal Ave.
Baltimore, MD 21217
301-225-9400
800-638-2300
TDD (for the deaf): 301-225-9409

SPORTS VISION

National Academy of Sports Vision
200 S. Progress Ave.
Harrisburg, PA 17109
717-652-8080

VISION THERAPY

College of Optometrists in Vision Development
P.O. Box 285
Chula Vista, CA 92010
619-425-6191

Optometric Extension Program Foundation
2912 S. Daimler St.
Santa Ana, CA 92705
714-250-8070

MISCELLANEOUS

American Academy of Ophthalmology
655 Beach St.
P.O. Box 7424
San Francisco, CA 94120-7424
415-561-8500

American Optometric Association
243 N. Lindbergh Blvd.
St. Louis, MO 63141
314-991-4100

Downing Institute
Brain science research
2261 Market St., Suite 504
San Francisco, CA 94114
415-626-0083

Eye Bank Association of America, Inc.
1511 K St., NW, Suite 830
Washington, DC 20005-1401
202-628-4280

National Academy of Opticianry
10111 Martin Luther King, Jr. Highway, Suite 112
Bowie, MD 20720
301-577-4828

Suggested Reading

Hyman, J. W. *The Light Book: How Natural and Artificial Light Affect Our Health, Mood and Behavior*. Los Angeles: Jeremy P. Tarcher, 1990.

Kavner, R. and L. Duskey. *Total Vision*. New York: A&W Publishers, 1978.

Kirschmann, J. D. and L. J. Dunne. *Nutrition Almanac*. 2d ed. New York: McGraw-Hill, 1984.

The Medicine Show. Compiled by the editors of *Consumer Reports*. Mount Vernon, NY: Consumers Union, 1980.

Rosenberg, H. *The Book of Vitamin Therapy*. New York: G. P. Putnam's Sons, 1980.

Seiderman, A. S. and S. E. Marcus. *20/20 Is Not Enough*. New York: Alfred A. Knopf, 1989.

Wertenbaker, L. *The Eye: Window To The World*. Washington, DC: U. S. News Books, Human Body Series, 1981.

Bibliography

Ayres, A. J. *Sensory Integration and Learning Disorders.* Los Angeles: Western Psychological Services, 1972.

Davson, H. *Physiology of the Eye.* 3d ed. London: Academic Press, 1972.

Fraunfelder, F. T. *Drug-Induced Ocular Side Effects and Drug Interactions.* Philadelphia: Lea & Febiger, 1976.

Getman, G. N. *How To Develop Your Child's Intelligence.* 7th ed. Wayne, PA: Research Publications, 1962.

Getman, G. N. and A. Gesell. *Vision: Its Development in Infant and Child.* New York: Harper & Row, 1949.

Glasspool, M. *Eyes: Their Problems and Treatments.* New York: Arco Publishing, 1984.

Goldberg, S. *Ophthalmology Made Ridiculously Simple.* 3d ed. Miami, FL: MedMaster, 1986.

Gregory, R. L. *Eye and Brain: The Psychology of Seeing.* London: World University Library, 1966.

Hyman, J. W. *The Light Book: How Natural and Artificial Light Affect Our Health, Mood and Behavior.* Los Angeles: Jeremy P. Tarcher, 1990.

Maciocia, G. *The Foundations of Chinese Medicine.* New York: Churchill Livingston, 1989.

Mitchell, H. S., H. J. Rynbergen, L. Anderson and M. V. Dibble. *Nutrition in Health and Disease.* 16th ed. Philadelphia: J. B. Lippincott, 1976.

Moses, R. A. *Adler's Physiology of the Eye—Clinical Application.* 5th ed. St. Louis: C.V. Mosby, 1970.

O'Conner, J. and D. Bensky, translators. *Acupuncture: A Comprehensive Text.* Chicago: Eastland Press, 1981.

Paraquin, C. A. *Eye Teasers.* 6th ed. New York: Sterling Publications, 1982.

Parks, M. M. *Atlas of Strabismus Surgery.* New York: Harper & Row, 1983.

Pearson, D. and S. Shaw. *Life Extension.* New York: Warner Books, 1982.

Roper-Hall, M.J. *Stallard's Eye Surgery.* 7th ed. London: Butterworth Scientific, 1989.

Weiner, M.A. *Earth Medicine, Earth Foods: Plant Remedies, Drugs, and Natural Foods of the North American Indians.* New York and London: Collier and Collier-Macmillan, 1972.

Wold, R. M., editor. *Vision: Its Impact on Learning.* Chula Vista, CA: Special Child Publications, 1978.

About the Author

Jeffrey Anshel, O.D., graduated from the Illinois College of Optometry in 1975. Dr. Anshel served in the United States Navy, where he established a vision therapy clinic, from 1975 to 1977. In 1978, he began practicing alternative eye care, including nutritional counseling, vision therapy, color therapy and acupressure.

In 1984, he opened a general optometric practice in Cardiff, California, where he combined traditional with alternative vision care. He opened a second office in Del Mar, California, in 1988. In the past, he has served on the staff of the Santa Fe College of Natural Medicine in Santa Fe, New Mexico.

Dr. Anshel is the author of several articles on the influence of nutrition on vision and on stress factors that affect vision. He now lives in La Costa, California, with his wife, Elaine, and their two children.

Contributors and Consultants

Technical Consultants

James A. Parks, O.D.
Tucson, Arizona
Richard A. Wahl, M.D.
Tucson, Arizona

Editor

Margaret Wahl
Tucson, Arizona

Illustrators

Joe Gherardini
Solana Beach, California
Ed Powers
Los Angeles, California
Randy Summerlin
Tucson, Arizona

Index